Neuroses

and Personality

Disorders

ELTON B. McNEIL

Prentice-Hall, Inc., Englewood Cliffs, New Jersey

Library of Congress Catalog Card Number 70–131382

Printed in the United States of America

Current Printing (last digit):

10 9 8 7 6 5 4 3 2 1

PRENTICE-HALL INTERNATIONAL, INC., London
PRENTICE-HALL OF AUSTRALIA, PTY. LTD., Sydney
PRENTICE-HALL OF CANADA, LTD., Toronto
PRENTICE-HALL OF INDIA PRIVATE LIMITED, New Delhi
PRENTICE-HALL OF JAPAN, INC., Tokyo

Contents

*Neuroses
and Personality
Disorders*

THE NEUROSES *I*

The Nature of
Neurosis

1

What kinds of difficulties bring people to a clinical psychologist or psychiatrist?

A SAMPLER OF ABERRANT
BEHAVIOR

—A bright and attractive 27 year old woman has become increasingly concerned about her sexually promiscuous behavior. Her inability to say "No" makes her feel guilty and unclean, but she is obsessed with sexual thoughts during most of her waking hours.

—A young housewife is preoccupied with thoughts of death and cannot be reassured despite a number of medical examinations. When each physician gives her a clean bill of health, she recalls that "some people walk out of the doctor's office and fall dead in the street."

—An ex-soldier ritualistically organizes his life to avoid contact with dirt and germs. He does not touch doorknobs and holds his breath when passing a hospital.

—At a time when energetic attention to his work is most needed, a middle-aged businessman finds himself lethargic and unable to concentrate.

—An accountant whose life was always exceptionally well-organized, abandoned his family and assumed a new identity in another town. Identified months later, he is unable to recall his previous way of life.

—Following the death of her father, a young woman became blind,

3

mute, and unable to feel anything in her limbs. No organic disturbance is discovered to account for these symptoms, and she seems quite unperturbed about her physical catastrophe.

Human behaviors of these kinds are most often labeled psychoneuroses or neurotic reactions. Psychoneurosis is an emotional disturbance characterized by severe anxiety or exaggerated defensive attempts to ward off anxiety. The neurotic individual's personality is not grossly disorganized and he does not usually require hospitalization. Neurosis is a disturbance of opposites and overreactions: phobic persons who cannot touch a doorknob and those who must obsessively touch it six times before turning it, persons who cannot leave the house while others cannot tolerate a shut-in feeling, and those who shun water while others cannot stop bathing. These persons are not sick in a medical sense. There is no disease present to account for their disturbances.

Disorder and Adjustment

Ideally, difficulties and conflicts of the sort described should be solved realistically by considering the essential elements of the problem and working out a rational plan of remedial action. Persons experiencing neurotic reactions, unfortunately, seem unable to see accurately all the components of their conflict, fail to function efficiently enough to work out a solution, or may use problem-solving methods which are inappropriate. For example, most people have some difficulty relating to an authority figure who is overbearing, too directive, or unsympathetic. If one must work or live with such an authority figure, responses such as a noncontroversial attitude, carrying out distasteful directives in a spirit of cooperation while disguising one's irritation, or resorting consciously to flattery may be realistic, if ignoble, solutions to the problem. The neurotic, however, overreacts by becoming argumentative, provocative, competitive, challenging, or openly derogatory. He may, by his responses, intensify the problem rather than solve it.

Workable solutions to interpersonal problems are "adjustments" in which the individual, unable to modify the demands being made on him, internally alters his feelings and thoughts or changes his overt response in such a way that the problem is no longer a significant issue in his life. Understanding the adjustment process is vital to our comprehension of the neuroses and personality disorders.

All living organisms tend to maintain a state of physical and psychological consistency and balance. When this tranquil internal state is disturbed by biological deficiencies or needs, bodily mechanisms go into action until the provocative stimulus ceases to exist. Adjustment, thus, involves need satisfaction and tension reduction—the overcoming of social or physical obstacles to achieve a satisfactory relationship to the environment. In infrahuman species, adaptation behavior is thought to be limited by instinct. The building of homes by ants, the flying south of birds in winter, the swimming upstream of salmon to spawn are all examples of previously unpracticed performances which seem to be an innate part of the response repertoire of each member of the species.

Man lacks these built-in responses, but he is blessed with an enormous capacity for adaptation through learning, i.e., the calculated modification of his own behavior. An animal cannot adapt to environmental change even though its instinctive behavior may have fatal consequences. The greater flexibility of man's behavior is also, potentially, a greater source of inconsistency and conflict for him.

Adjustment is, at best, a complicated process that must be evaluated in relative rather than absolute terms. A pattern of response is adequate, effective, or "good" if it reduces regularly recurring internal tensions without unduly interfering with the satisfaction of other motives or with the adjustment of other people.

Since inner conflict (the clash of motives within the self) is the most salient characteristic of the neurotic state, the neurotic usually is ambivalent about what he wants and doesn't want and is attracted yet frightened by persons and situations. These conflicts may make him restless, unsatisfied, uneasy, depressed, pent-up, or bored. And unsatisfactory adjustments are made since some tensions are dealt with while significant others are not.

"NEUROSIS" IN ANIMALS

Studies of animal neuroses illustrate rather dramatically some of the central features of adjustment. Jules H. Masserman and others (1946) experimentally created neuroses in animals in the hope of gaining greater insight into man. Their method was simple. First, they put a very hungry cat in a glass cage and dropped food into a box with a hinged lid within the cage. A flashing light and a ringing bell signaled each feeding time. When the cat perceived this light-and-bell combination, it would rush to the box and lift the lid. Occasionally it was greeted by a powerful blast of compressed air and would react by rushing to the other end of the cage and crouching there, tensely. Hunger eventually drove the cat back to the box, and it learned that, in an unpredictable sequence, it was sometimes subjected to the traumatic, frightening air blast, while at other times it was simply provided with food and could eat without terror. After some days, the conflict between hunger and fear made the cat respond to the feeding signal itself with anxiety (tenseness, increased blood pressure and pulse rate, sudden urination or defecation). Previously placid cats became restless, agitated pacers, some became preoccupied with the self (cleaned and licked itself unceasingly and repeatedly invited petting and fondling), and some became vicious and quick to attack.

It is also possible to induce equally serious and lasting disordered behavior by forcing an animal to choose between two attractive but mutually exclusive satisfactions. For example, a hungry female cat in heat must choose between food and a male cat, or a hungry mother cat must decide between her own needs and the demands of a meowing litter needing milk. Such mutually exclusive positive motivations can engender severe anxiety, compulsive avoidance, or paralyzing depression. Normal animals, introduced to such disturbing circumstances, become indecisive, hesitant, and distractable; neurotic animals exposed continuously to such conflicts and problem situations, show even more severe abnormal behavior.

It is tempting, of course, to draw a series of direct parallels between the behavior of "neurotic" cats and the response to conflict of human beings. Thus, for example, "neurotic" cats with alcohol added to their milk will, suffused with alcoholic courage, approach the feeding box with an elegant disregard for any possible traumatic consequences. While this behavior may remind us of the meek and mild fighting drunk, the analogy is imperfect. Man is a more complicated animal and we must explore the unique human personality to comprehend the neuroses.

While this account of early studies of artificial neuroses induced in animals has a certain fascination in and by itself, we must ask how these comparative studies have assisted us in understanding the nature of human neuroses. The study of animals has the advantage of being objective, reliable, and describable in clear-cut terms, but it has the disadvantage of having limited applicability to the human condition. As Wolman (1965) observes, "One may or may not be convinced that what happened in experimental animals under stress was a neurosis" (p. 11). Most often, those who experiment with animals move glibly from observable fact to speculative theories about mental disorder, and the trustworthiness of their conclusions is suspect despite the absolute reliability of the facts from which these theories are construed. As Wolman examines the experimental work with animals he wonders whether all or any part of it applies to human beings. As he asks, "Would a man break down whenever he could not discriminate between a circle and an ellipse? Are happy-go-lucky, unambitious men who have no goal necessarily frustrated? Do they inevitably head toward a nervous breakdown?" (p. 11).

Thus, the logic of inferences from animal to man seldom bears up under scrutiny. Analogy remains a useful, thought-stimulating device but one subject to a host of logical errors. The best of animal studies cannot substitute for the direct study of man. Comparative studies are suggestive, but we must turn now to the more relevant studies of human disorders.

PERSONALITY DEVELOPMENT
AND NEUROSIS

Neurosis is not understandable apart from some theory of personality structure, development, and function. We will briefly outline some of Freud's views and premises about the psychic apparatus, the structure of personality, and the form of ego development since these issues are intimately connected to neurotic development and will provide part of the conceptual scaffolding needed to explain anxiety neurosis, depression, obsessive and compulsive reactions, hysteria, and phobia.

First, Freud assumed that all behavior is motivated, that there are triggering factors which set it into motion, and that it is generally purposeful. Second, he believed in strict psychological determinism, i.e., no behavior, feeling, or thought is accidental, fortuitous, or uncaused. Third, he assumed that an historical account of past life is needed to understand current behavior. Fourth, he used the concept of unconscious motivation as a means of explaining behavior for which the person himself often could not account.

Layers of Consciousness

Conscious experience contains those thoughts and feelings in the forefront of awareness and attention at any moment in time. Preconscious experience contains psychological contents and memories which, though not in the person's awareness at the moment, can be brought to awareness by an effort of will and attention. Thus, if you are asked who wrote Tom Sawyer you might respond with "Mark Twain" even though you were not *consciously* aware of that fact the moment before the question was asked.

Unconscious mental processes, however, are not capable of becoming conscious in this way. Through a process labeled repression, the psychic apparatus of each of us "arranges" to eliminate painful or unacceptable impulses, fantasies, or motives from consciousness. This self-protective psychic maneuver frees the individual from the distress of conscious anxiety, but this freedom proves to be a costly state to achieve. Ideally, each of us should deal directly with reality and solve its problems without recourse to self-deception. This ideal state is, however, reached by only a few very mature individuals.

The unconscious consists of drive states, motives, fantasies, and impulses which the individual cannot perceive directly but which nevertheless exercise a guiding influence on conscious behavior and feeling. The unconscious can only be inferentially revealed in slips of the tongue, dreams, faulty actions, and in the functional disturbances of the neuroses. To bring unconscious material into consciousness was Freud's first formula for dealing with the neurotic symptoms of his patients. Behind the symptom, Freud felt, lay a series of emotional events that the patient did not consciously perceive and often did not want to know.

The Structure of Personality

Freud subscribed to a genetic or developmental view of personality which stated that the individual is best understood as an organization of imperative, biologically based drives (needs) requiring periodic fulfillment and discharge to relieve tension. Before birth, the organism's needs are taken care of by automatic biological mechanisms; needs arise and are fulfilled without tension. After birth the child's needs are no longer automatically fulfilled and he is dependent on objects outside himself to provide food, liquids, warmth, dryness, moderate cleanliness, and appropriate stimulation. He also experiences a growing time lag between the onset of his needs and their gratification.

To this primary and basic part of the self (drives and needs which create tension and seek fulfillment), Freud gave the name *id*. The instincts of the id are described in terms of a number of characteristics they possess: (1) *Aim:* the aim of all instincts is gratification, satisfaction, and reduction of tension. (2) *Source:* all instincts derive from the organ system involved with the specific drive. With hunger, the digestive and circulatory systems are primarily involved; with sex, the genitals, certain glandular and hormonal systems, and some aspects of the central and autonomic nervous systems are involved. (3) *Object:* varies with regard to the drive involved. Food and water are objects of hunger and thirst drives. A variety of persons and objects may be the object of sex drives. (4) *Quantity:* refers to the intensity of the drive and may be a function of how much frustration the drive has undergone.

The id is governed by the *pleasure principle*. When organisms experience drives or needs, they seek only to relieve tension as soon as possible. The newborn infant, dominated by the id system, wants what he wants when he wants it. The personality of the infant at birth consists almost entirely of his group of drives or instincts striving for gratification or fulfillment. Birth exposes the infant to frustration and development pivots on this fact. If all his needs were taken care of immediately, the development of a psychological apparatus to arrange for independent self-gratification would not occur.

Soon, the sense organs of focused vision, auditory acuity, touch and temperature, smell and taste, locomotor balance, and spatial orientation will allow the child to perceive not only the goings-on around him but also the boundaries between himself and the environment outside himself. In the early months of life a child cannot make this distinction, and it is through experience that he begins to develop the notion that he is a distinct entity. His experiences with pain and pleasure and with alternate states of gratification and tension teach him that he depends for gratification on sources over which he has no immediate control.

To achieve independence, the child develops a psychic apparatus which Freud referred to as the *ego*. This part of personality is organized by the *principle of reality*. A growing child soon comprehends that if he fails to inhibit or direct his pleasure striving he will come into painful conflict with a dangerous environment. The child learns to restrict and delay his impulses in order to avoid punishment or disapproval and to assure his security, comfort, and survival. The goal of pleasure is not abandoned; it is tempered by reality, and danger is signaled by anxiety whenever the child's urges threaten to get him into a dangerous situation.

Human existence would surely be less complicated if the story of personality development were to end at this point, since life would contain no injunctions about right and wrong or good and bad; we would, rather, listen only to the limitations of feasible and not feasible. We could each eat when hungry, drink when dry, have sexual relations when the urge is strident, and live without shame, fear, guilt, or depression. Man is, however, a social animal and he finds it necessary to curb unbridled impulses with a complicated system of rules and regulations. The child learns of these limits as he grows and develops just as he learns to strive to emulate an ideal or model of proper behavior. In short, the child acquires a *super ego*—a psychic apparatus that makes him feel anxious when he violates social rules and expectations for behavior just as it makes him anxious if he fails to achieve a style of life that matches the ideal represented by significant figures in his early life. Violations of the proscriptions of the super ego produce anxiety that plays a major role in the development of neurotic rather than normal reactions to conflict. To complete this explanation of neurosis formation, we must describe the defense mechanisms the psychic apparatus devises to ease the pain of anxiety.

The Defense Mechanisms

The rewards and punishments meted out to the growing child by parents force him both to control the behavior he displays to others and to wash his mind clean of those thoughts and impulses he has learned are not approved by others. To make clear how the child learns to defend himself against anxiety we can use love and hate as an illustration.

. . . The most casual observation would reveal that when the mother spanks the child, deprives him of things he desires, or interferes with his attempts at gratification of his needs, the child, at least at that moment, hates his mother and has powerful aggressive urges directed toward her. The society insists that such hostile feelings have no place in the mother-child relationship and that the child must be free of such emotions if he is to be accepted and loved by his mother and to feel worthwhile as a person. At this point the child faces a conflict he must resolve, and he comes to learn that a number of avenues are open to him, although each will be less satisfactory than being able to accept his impulses and feelings as a normal consequence of human existence. Thus the child must learn to manipulate his feelings if he is to defend himself against the onslaught of unbearable anxiety.

How can the child avoid being caught, by himself or others, with contraband feelings? There are four elements or dimensions of the forbidden situation that he can alter to bring about a new situation more in keeping with society's dictates and his own anxieties. Momentarily, he feels that he hates his mother and wants to kill her. There is the source (himself) of the feeling, the impulse (hate), the object (mother) toward which it is directed, and the aim (kill) of the impulse. Alteration of any one of these aspects will produce a formula which is no longer threatening to his self-esteem or to the esteem others have for him. He can, for example, change the *source* in some fashion and not tamper with the other elements; now *he* doesn't hate his mother and want to kill her. Or he can alter the *impulse* so that he *loves* his mother, not hates her. The *object* can be transformed so that he hates *school* but not his mother. Another compromise that will solve his dilemma is to admit that he hates his mother but merely wishes to *reprimand* her rather than kill her. In each instance, a slight change in his perception of the reality of hating his mother cleans up the thought and makes it presentable. In extreme circumstances the whole thought must be changed, leaving no element unaltered; in less threatening situations it is necessary only to reduce the intensity of each element of the sequence. This means that the kind, quality, and degree of distortion will always be dependent upon the demands made by the environment and the internal psychic resources he has available to him. In one family a child must see, hear, speak, and think no evil, while in another an aggressive outburst is a natural event which must be managed but is viewed as a reasonable consequence of the frustrations of living with other people.

At first, mechanisms for managing hostile feelings are practiced in a conscious form by the child. He will, for example, retain his feelings but suppress the overt attack on the mother to insure her continued acceptance of him. Such feelings, as well as the act of altering a prohibited situation, must be hidden from both the self and others (after all, the best-adjusted adult could not be comfortable thinking murderous thoughts about others all day). Through a process we can label, but not fully understand, the effort that the child once made willfully and consciously becomes an event which occurs in so subtle a fashion that no one is the wiser.

This description of perceptual maneuvering to escape experiencing anxiety is particularly relevant to aggressive impulses which, because of their potential destructiveness, must be highly regulated and controlled. The average person in our society is made quite uncomfortable by the sight of naked hostility in himself or in others, since one of the hallmarks of maturity is control over aggression. The description of the need to defend one's self makes it appear that this is a consciously willed, mechanical process—something like a bag of tricks used when appropriate to the emergency. A more apt description would be that normal persons *cope* with frustrations and forbidden impulses and only *defend* against them when no other alternative remains. When defensive tactics relieve anxiety, this very relief will reinforce the defensive behavior and tend to solidify it into a habitual and characteristic pattern of reaction when faced with conflict in the future. When this occurs, they no longer act as emergency reactions but become predictable character traits that distinguish the individual for life. Since a variety of defense mechanisms is available to the individual, he usually proceeds by trial-and-error to select those that are the most effective in freeing him from guilt and anxiety. A mechanism that proves to be effective in one situation is tried in another and its use continued until it fails to accomplish its purpose. Highly flexible individuals may acquire a set of defenses which are adapted specifically to each situation; rigid or less resourceful persons may become general defenders who find one dramatic mechanism that works (such as thoroughgoing repression) and use it for a variety of situations and with all kinds of impulses.

Using hostility as the model of impulses to be dealt with, what are the ways in which it can be managed defensively? At a broad level, the choices of the individual are restricted to *changing the situation* through the process of conscious problem-solving and working out a new relationship with the person toward whom he is hostile; *escaping from the situation* by running away or retreating into a fantasy life where the problems do not exist, or *changing his perception of the hostile situation* through defense mechanisms which render it innocuous (McNeil, 1959; pp. 210–11).

The Meaning of Neurosis

The psychic distortions of reality implied by the defense mechanisms constitute the core issue in neurosis and make comprehensible the seemingly irrational aspects of behavior we label neurotic. We can proceed now to examine the symptom patterns produced by such defensive efforts to ward off anxiety. The American Psychiatric Association has developed a widely-used but imperfect set of diagnostic categories to describe psychoneurotic reactions. These disorders are considered to be of psychogenic origin, i.e., disorders not clearly or tangibly attributable to structural or bodily diseases:

PSYCHONEUROTIC REACTIONS

Anxiety reaction
Dissociative reaction
Conversion reaction
Phobic reaction
Obsessive-compulsive reaction
Depressive reaction

Despite the clear disclaimer that the psychoneuroses are not classic, organic illnesses, this diagnostic and nosological system implies that we are dealing with a disease—a disease rather than a disorder of living.

From a strictly medical point of view, all disorder implies disease, but in recent years a different conception of neurosis has come to the fore.

Stated simply and directly, a great many modern theorists are convinced that the psychological difficulties we label neuroses are treated professionally as though they were physical disorders rather than problems of living in a complex society. Earlier, we defined the psychoneuroses as emotional disturbances characterized by severe anxiety or exaggerated defensive attempts to ward off anxiety. This definition would suggest, logically, that some form of psychological reconstruction or repair would be an appropriate remedy. Yet, year by year, we escalate the rate at which we drug emotionally disturbed persons rather than deal with the underlying psychological causes.

What modern-day theorists are suggesting is that the entire form, style, and means of treatment of the disorders of living might better have a psychological rather than a medical model as a guide. These theorists insist that the historical definition of emotional difficulties as medical problems has unfortunately led us down a theoretical blind alley.

Suppose, for example, neurosis and psychosis were viewed merely as differing degrees of conscious, personal eccentricity chosen by the individual as a style of life? Would you drug him, shock him, operate on his brain, or confine him to an institution in order to cure his socially unacceptable way of living and relating to others? Some theorists have then concluded that our professional and social response to emotional disturbance has been to treat it "as though" it was an event identical to being diabetic, suffering a breakdown of the nervous system, or being afflicted with polio. As a consequence, these theorists insist we have failed utterly to understand the nature of human emotional disorder.

Sanford (1958) argues, for example, that we have long suffered from an erroneous orientation to the pathological and an exclusive focus on the clinical to the extent that we have erected an invisible barrier to exploration of much of the adaptive, creative, resilient, spontaneously inventive, and consummately human behavior of which man is capable. Thomas Szasz (1960) said it in a different fashion in an article entitled "The Myth of Mental Illness." Szasz, a psychiatrist and psychoanalyst, expressed serious dissatisfaction with the vague, capricious, generally inaccurate nature of the concept of mental illness. According to Szasz, although most of the observations in the field of abnormal psychology and clinical psychiatry are couched in medical-psychiatric terms, these observations are most often of patterns of human behavior and human communication gleaned from listening to and talking with patients. In contrast, the conceptual scaffolding of medicine rests on the principles of physics and chemistry rather than interpersonal communication. Man's sign-using behavior, his problems in interpersonal relations, and his social difficulties in adjustment do not lend themselves to exploration and understanding in purely medical terms.

The term "mental illness" is still widely used despite the fact that most personality theory is psychological and social rather than biological and medical. Much of psychotherapy revolves around the elucidation and weighing of goals and values and the means whereby they might best be harmonized, realized, or relinquished. The concept of mental illness underemphasizes conflicting human needs, values, and aspirations by providing an amoral and impersonal "thing" (an "illness") as the explanation for *problems in living*. In our review of the neuroses it is important to keep in mind that there is a growing disaffection with a purely medical conception of these disorders and a beginning attempt to define neurotic reactions in psychological and social terms.

From an historical point of view it is not surprising that neurosis came to be viewed in medical rather than psychological terms. The earliest scientific views of emotional or mental disorders were cast almost exclusively in terms of diseases of the brain. This somatogenic hypothesis maintained that the genesis of troubled psychological behavior would, one day, be traced to some measurable disorder in the body. The millenium would occur when the brain and human constitution disgorged their long-hidden secrets and, at that moment, we would solve the riddle of disordered thought and behavior. This organic viewpoint was reinforced by the elaborate medical detective work that uncovered a physical basis for the disordered behavior that accompanied general paresis. Theorists in those days observed that the discovery of a physical basis for one puzzling disorder augered well for similar revelations in the future for all disorders.

In 1798, the physician Haslam observed a group of patients suffering a general paralysis marked by delusions of grandeur and disturbance of logical thought processes. This physical and psychological disturbance not only followed a typical and predictable course, it regularly had a fatal outcome. In a majority of these cases, two abnormalities were present: a diminished pupillary reflex (the Argyll-Robertson pupil) and an exaggerated patella-tendon reflex (the knee jerk). Both signs pointed to a disorder of the central nervous system and, on autopsy, evidence accumulated indicating such patients had microscopically damaged cortical areas of the brain. Nearly 100 years after Haslam's observations, Fournier uncovered the fact that a history of syphilis infection was present in nearly 65 percent of such paretic patients. Even though 35 percent of the cases failed to confirm the theory, a great theoretical leap was taken and it was hypothesized that syphilis was the prime source of brain damage which, in turn, evoked motor disturbance (behavioral paralysis) and thought disturbance (grandiosity and dementia). The unaccounted for 35 percent, theorists reasoned, may have, for conscious or unconscious reasons, lied about or forgotten those socially unacceptable sexual adventures of their youth that could have given them syphilis infections.

It was Kraft-Ebbing, in 1897, who conducted a daring and probably unethical test of this early theory. He injected blood taken from known syphilitic patients into the veins of seven paretic persons who had steadfastly denied the possibility of encounter with syphilis. It was a frightening gamble. If those patients, who denied sexual adventuring in their life, were indeed unexposed previously to syphilis infection, the experimental innoculation would certainly have insured an infection, and there was, at that time in history, no cure for the disease. Fortunately, none of the paretic patients developed signs of syphilitic infection; they were immune to the innoculation. This risky experiment provided irrefutable proof that patients suffering paresis *must* have been infected with the syphilis spirochete at some time in the past and had, consequently, developed an immunity to reinfection.

By 1905, advances in laboratory techniques allowed scientists to examine the cerebrospinal fluid of paretic patients. In their spinal fluid was found the minute organism *treponema pallidum* known to be the cause of syphilis. Shortly thereafter, Noguchi and Moore traced the syphilis organism to the nerve cells of the brain and the essential cause of paresis was once and for all revealed. The magnificence of this single but outstanding instance of scientific detective work was used, again and again, to bolster scientific hopes that one day all emotional and behavioral disorders would reveal their roots in human physiology.

This brief detective story about the discovery of an organic basis for the psychological complications of paresis is recounted here simply to point up a moral relevant to the issue of a disease versus disorder-in-living explanation of mental "illness." Those who view emotional disturbance as a psychological and social event do not deny that human beings have bodies. Nor do they maintain that tissue or nervous system damage is not reflected in disorganization or disorder in the psychological life of the individual. What they do insist upon, however, is that these biological sources of distress be placed in a reasonable and proper perspective and not be used as the sole explanation of human emotional disturbance. Use of a medical, biological, organic model for the understanding of mankind's troubles is not only inaccurate, it is misleading in that it promotes the tendency to evade the primary problems of living by attributing disorder to organic malfunction.

SUMMARY

A variety of distortions of human existence are labeled neurotic, but they constitute only special cases of the attempt of an individual to adjust to the pressures and anxieties of living. Animals confronted with unresolvable conflict will display neurotic-like behavior, but man's complicated psychic apparatus requires a more complex theory of the sources of neurotic reactions. To comprehend disorder in human life we must refer to layers of consciousness, the structure of personality (the id, ego, and super ego), and the defensive psychic maneuvers man is capable of in his quest to escape the unbearable onslaught of anxiety. Although it was a natural and understandable progression from early medical concern with "physical" illness to the current conception of "mental" illness, theorists have begun to examine the possibility that neurosis might more fruitfully be defined as a learned, social, and psychological disorder of living rather than an "illness" in the classic sense.

Anxiety Reactions

Theorists of a psychogenic persuasion insist that how one manages anxiety is fundamental to the development of a psychoneurosis. The psychic techniques employed to reduce or avoid anxiety become the hallmarks of neurosis and determine, in great part, the pattern of symptoms the neurotic individual will display. As man attempts to deal with anxiety, he fashions a style of life that comes to distinguish him from others.

The anxious person reacts in typical ways in our society, i.e., he may begin to display somatic symptoms that have no basis in organic malfunctioning, he may react excessively to objects and situations that most of us treat in a casual fashion, or he may be frightened perpetually by a daily life that holds more terror than pleasure. Anxiety is an exaggerated fear reaction; the anxious individual is afraid of things others don't fear, anticipates a host of possible future threats to his well-being, and has little or no insight into why he is such a frightened person.

Some theoretical explication about anxiety is necessary since, according to classic Freudian psychoanalytic views, there are both *actual neuroses* and *psychoneuroses*.

When forbidden id impulses seek expression and provoke crippling anxiety, repressive attempts to eliminate the impulse from consciousness may be necessary. If the repressed impulses are adequately managed by this psychic maneuver (as they may have been in early childhood) all may be well even though a costly state of tension is the price paid for the absence of anxiety. This bottling-up of repressed impulses produces symptoms (fatigue, emotional instability, pain) most accurately attributed to an actual neurosis. Such a neurosis may be delineated by anxiety that

17

is free-floating (not tied specifically to an object, person, or situation) and characteristic of the individual's style of life.

When simple repression fails (as it may in adolescence, for example, when biological changes increase the strength of sexual impulses) the ego must defend itself more vigorously against the anxiety produced by the reappearance in consciousness of unacceptable impulses. The defense mechanisms used by the ego to ward off anxiety produce behavior that is labeled psychoneurotic, and the kinds of defenses necessary to quell anxiety determine the form of psychoneurosis that will mark the individual's life. The imperfectly repressed impulse finds its way to conscious expression but in a distorted and disguised form that does not provoke anxiety.

Actual neuroses are thus characterized by a continued tenseness, energy-expenditure, and irritability occasioned by massive repression. And they are underscored, at times, by brief attacks of acute panic when impulses accidentally break through. This chronic restlessness and tension is tied closely to continuing apprehension that some forbidden impulse will break out of psychic confinement in raw form and provoke anxiety. The individual is not consciously aware that this is his problem; he experiences only tension, fatigue, depression, or excessive concern about a suspected failing state of physical health. If repression is the only workable defense, anxiety can pervade every facet of its victim's life as he is whipsawed between the expression of the impulse and the fear of punishment for so doing.

When forbidden impulses move closer than usual to expression, panic may result. In the explosive outburst that follows there may be some venting of the impulse (catharsis) which produces a new, temporary equilibrium between impulse and repression. The legendary prohibitionist, Carrie Nation, for example, must have felt sublime satisfaction and relief from tension as she and her coworkers demolished local saloons while striking a blow against the Demon Rum. Normal persons, of course, have many of the same conflicts that plague neurotics. As Buss (1966) has noted, however, neurotics have conflicts of greater intensity and seek relief from anxiety in more primitive ways—ways better fitted to earlier and less complicated stages of life.

Those who must repress rather than cope rationally with unacceptable impulses have little psychic energy to devote to other social or interpersonal enterprises. And if there is a subtle awareness of the touch-and-go repressive contest being waged internally, the outcome can only be depression. We will speak of depression at greater length later; it will be sufficient at this juncture to note that those suffering anxiety reactions

go out, though, and tip-toed over to the edge without looking down. I closed my eyes and clung to the balustrade but I still began to feel dizzy. The worst part of it was not the possibility that I might faint and fall over the edge, it was the terrible urge I felt to run to the barrier, jump, and kill myself. It was like the Sword of Damocles that hung by a thread over the head of the King. I found myself thinking it would be better to jump and get it over with than to worry that I would fall by accident. When we got back to the pavement I was so shaky I started to cry but I couldn't tell Jim what it was all about.

Caroline's frightening experience took place on her honeymoon in New York. She could recall no other time in her life when she had undergone quite so violent an upheaval triggered by height alone (McNeil, 1967; p. 62).

Few of us are without anxiety confronted by the prospect of teetering precariously on the parapet of a 10-storey building. Yet, not many among us are so petrified with fear at just the *thought* of such heights. And not many among us are obsessed with the impulse to leap over the edge to relieve the tension of the situation. We learn of the fear and pain of falling early in life but these facts of life do not dominate our whole existence. For those phobic about heights, the fear of falling encompasses the entirety of their personal and social life.

The anxiety reflected in the encounter with a dreaded object is anxiety displaced from its proper object and attached, instead, to some symbolic equivalent that stands in its place. In the classic psychodynamic explanation of phobia, for example, it would be necessary to trace the inordinate fear of heights experienced by Caroline W. to some source other than the realistic danger present. This search for reasons might take us on a journey through the patient's natural history to study the way in which basic lessons of impulse control were learned early in life in order to untangle the twisting path by which anxiety got displaced to an object outside the self.

Phobic reactions are most usual among young, near-adult females. The incidence of acknowledged phobia among males would undoubtedly be higher were it not for strict cultural standards that define courage and bravery as essential facets of the masculine role. It is acceptably feminine in our society to shrink from terrifying situations; it is masculine to face danger squarely. Phobias not only reveal cultural definitions of proper secondary characteristics of men and women, they also reflect the degree of technical sophistication of the society. Kerry (1960), for example, reported four patients who had intense phobias centering on outer space; they were anxious about residing on a planet that, like a gigantic space ship, hurtled through space at an incredible speed.

Most phobias are less exotic, of course. Dixon (1957) and his coworkers made statistical groupings of phobic responses reported by patients and concluded such symptoms could be grouped into two categories: fear of separation and fear of harm. Persons phobic about being left alone, being in the dark, or taking journeys are anxious, primarily, about interpersonal relations. Those whose fears are focused on harm (surgery, hospitals, or pain) share the common fears of most of us but the intensity of their reaction refers most directly to developmental experiences that have been inadequate to provide the maturity needed to face the harsh realities of life.

The Phobias of Childhood

Phobia has been described as the "neurosis of childhood" since it seems an inescapable part of growing up in a frightening and realistically dangerous world. The fears of childhood are also the terrors that come alive in later years to plague adult life. A recent selective review of the scientific literature on phobia during the last 40 years lists 300 articles devoted to this topic alone (Berecz, 1968).

Despite popular views to the contrary, the fears of childhood are learned less often by direct, immediate experience than by a process of "absorption" of the anxieties of grown-ups on whom children are dependent. Nervous parents produce nervous children; an apprehensive mother can communicate a generalized anxious state to the child even if the source of this fright is not spelled out. Children early in life react to the calm or agitated state of their parents, and it is impossible to specify that point in time when parental anxieties first find reflection in the feelings, attitudes, and behaviors of children. We suspect, however, it begins earlier than most of us believe.

The frightened child approaches challenges (separation from the parents, meeting strangers, or essaying new tasks) with a built-in reluctance and hesitation that may well determine whether he will succeed or fail in each new enterprise (Olsen and Coleman, 1967). Approaching new problems with dread and anticipation of failure must vitiate the child's effort to cope. Those free of anxiety are unable to empathize fully with the fearful, worried, nervous few in our society. The course of childhood differs remarkably for different persons and makes each of us incapable of comprehending the behavior of the other.

Phobic anxiety can have several sources. It can be of the contagious variety (learned from parents or others), it can be acquired via trauma (the frightening dog that barks and bites), or it can be the outcome of an internal psychic conflict that goes unresolved in childhood. It is this last possibility that is most relevant to our consideration of anxiety reactions that become focused (often only symbolically) on particular objects in the real world. The issue of phobic anxiety is deceptive, however. It is difficult to disentangle this mixture of traumatic experience, contagious learning, and symbolic representation in phobic persons when searching for the source of the problem.

It is conceivable, for example, that a phobic individual could have been traumatized by a painful experience with heights and have a mother with a morbid dread of high places yet react as he does for neither of these reasons. The traumatic experience and contagious learning might be the apparent rather than real reason for the person's exceptionally anxious reaction to heights.

The diagnostic and therapeutic issue is further complicated by the question of why some events are traumatic and others not. Some fears are acquired at the same moment that immunity exists for equally devastating terrors. How fears come into existence and why some persist remain only partly answered questions.

Managing Phobia

One way to deal with phobic feelings is to take defensive counterphobic measures rather than avoid the feared object. The phobic person can consciously and deliberately seek mastery of what he fears in order to deny to himself and others the truth of the anxiety that nibbles at the edge of his consciousness. Children regularly "act out" frightening situations (the dentist, the doctor) the better to manage them. And, in much the same way, adults indulge vigorously in precisely those behaviors that are most dreaded even though they may be unaware of the source of the fascination with such actions. Cameron (1963) describes this as a form of "reactive courage." Those who fear heights may climb mountains, those who fear speed may drive racing cars, and those who suffer from claustrophobia may devote their lives to spelunking—exploring caves.

This is not to suggest that the heros and dare-devils of our culture are all emotionally disturbed, obsessively counterphobic human beings. It is merely a way of noting that for some people dangerous acts are a means of demonstrating a mastery of certain fears. Thus, some skydivers are normal while others are attempting to compensate for neurotic problems.

Counterphobic behavior appears to be the precise opposite of the anxiety laden avoidance that usually characterizes the phobic. Dynamically they are closely related, however, since the counterphobic attempts to master his anxiety by compulsively and repetitively forcing himself into a confrontation with the phobic experience. The counterphobic, however, may appear no more anxious than most of us in the same situation since he is not consciously aware that there is a driven quality to his behavior —he climbs perilous mountains not because they are there but because conquering them is a symbolic mastery of anxieties he cannot understand or acknowledge. The counterphobic is a neurotic who has employed an additional, sophisticated defensive barrier in his attempt to deal with basic anxieties established early in his life. The activities of the counterphobic can never free him from the bondage of unconscious anxiety since he is solving the wrong problem—the mountain is nothing more than a symbolic representation of fears displaced from unconscious, forbidden impulses and tendencies.

Anthony (1967) observed that many of the phobic symptoms of childhood disappear in adults with or without treatment. Parents and teachers who encounter such natural fears tend to "shout down" these childish anxieties without awareness of the possible psychological and developmental impact such actions may have. Phobia can be eliminated, i.e., cease to appear in the child's overt behavior in response to a child's being shamed by adults or through his being forced into unwelcome confrontations with the fearsome stimuli, but we are not yet certain whether or not such symptom disappearance may trigger a chain of new compromises that are costly to the individual's psychological well-being even if deemed more acceptable socially.

The dilemma for the parent or teacher is in detecting which of the multitude of childhood fears is intractably rooted in neurotic conflict and thus ill served by repressive attempts at abolition and which of the fears can be eliminated through adequate emotional support, education, and development of personal skills. Psychological theorists are unable to provide a simple formula that will make this distinction clear. Theorists are currently embroiled in a heated disagreement among themselves about the origin, dynamics, and preferred remedy for childhood phobia.

Phobia and Therapy

When phobic behavior in children is severe and incapacitating it is often dealt with by traditional psychotherapeutic means coupled with active involvement of the parents in shaping the child's behavior (Andrews, 1966). In school phobia, for example, the therapist may probe for the meaning of the avoidance behavior and offer support and reassurance to the anxious child, yet compel the child to attend school, even if the experience is painful, since, if the child's phobic behavior succeeds, i.e., he is allowed to avoid school, the task of undoing the fundamental fear increases over time (Levanthal, Weinberger, Standler, and Stearns, 1967).

Most recently, the problems of dealing with phobia have been approached with some success by a new breed of behavioral therapists (Kennedy, 1965). Behavioral therapists reject customary psychiatric descriptive devices and speak of phobia as no more than an acquired habit of responding with fear to various stimuli present in the environment. These habits are considered nonadaptive, since they interfere with the normal conduct of life. Thus, fear and phobia become indistinguishable responses (except in terms of intensity) and their treatment, according to Wolpe (1967), no more complex than establishing a systematic program of desensitizing the child to the feared object or situation.

The therapeutic technique of desensitization involves repeatedly exposing the individual to objects or situations similar to those that are known to produce the phobic response. Beginning with exposure to stimuli that produce a very low level of anxiety, over time the intensity of exposure is increased by minute degrees until the phobic person can fearlessly face the situation that originally evoked a panicked response. Thus, for example, a person who dreads snakes may be desensitized in tiny steps beginning with a piece of a tiny, dead worm and culminating in the comfortable manipulation of large, lively snakes.

Research studies appraising the method of desensitization in treating phobic patients have recorded an astonishing degree of therapeutic effectiveness. Gelder and Marks (1968), for example, selected seven phobic patients who had failed to respond to long-term, traditional group psychotherapy and exposed them to desensitization procedures. They reported that, on the average, phobias improved three times more in four months of such treatment than they had in the previous two years of group psychotherapy. There is an additional report (Kahn and Baker, 1968) of sixteen phobic persons assigned randomly to desensitization procedures conducted in the laboratory and a similar "do-it-yourself" program of desensitization conducted by patients themselves at home. Using subjective reports of success as a measuring device, they reported both groups did equally well.

In the past, analytic theory has insisted that other symptoms would simply be substituted for the phobia if defensive fears were removed without regard for the underlying, dynamic function of such fears. This seems not to be the case, however, according to the preliminary evidence provided by behavioral therapists. Findings such as these suggest the need for a critical reevaluation of our traditional psychodynamic views of the varieties of phobia and their treatment. Behavioral therapists have had their most noteworthy therapeutic successes with these fairly-well delineated, circumscribed disorders. And they have alleviated fears and phobias without recourse to exploration of the source of the patient's anxiety. Their therapeutic methods are basically a-historical—they deal exclusively with the present—and variants of their primary techniques are being employed by a mushrooming number of practitioners of this general persuasion. Desensitization therapy for fears and phobias was practiced scientifically as early as 1924 (Jones, 1924) in removing a young child's fear of rabbits. The recent popularity of this approach has a firm base in the unmistakable success of the active approach to fears that once seemed treatable only with prolonged "insight" therapy (Paul, 1966). If fears and phobias can truly be alleviated simply by the methods of behavioral therapists it would be a boon to all. Some very practical social problems might be solved—pilots who are unable to fly high-performance jet aircraft, for example, might be able to complete training (Reinhart, 1967)—and the ordinary terrors each of us is secretly ashamed of might be made less frightening.

DISSOCIATIVE REACTIONS

A dissociative reaction is an unconscious attempt to manage anxiety which results in a form of personality disorganization that is distinguished by an alteration of the usual conscious state. As Kolb (1968) notes, "At times anxiety may so overwhelm and disorganize the personality that certain aspects or functions of it become dissociated from each other. In some instances, the personality may be so disorganized that defense mechanisms govern consciousness, memory, and temporarily even the total individual, with little or no participation on the part of the conscious personality" (p. 469).

According to psychoanalytic theory, dissociative reactions involve not only disturbances of memory but loss of awareness of personal identity. These reactions seem not to have received the attention from analytic theorists that, perhaps, they deserve. Dissociative reactions are dramatic but fairly rare since their appearance relies more heavily on the massive, pervasive use of the defense mechanism of repression than does any other neurosis. Again, infantile sexual impulses may be the original, repressed focus of anxiety that has unsuccessfully been sublimated and thus remains an active force in personality. When repression begins to break down, the individual regresses and acts out a wish-fulfilling fantasy which in turn produces even more anxiety and forces a splitting-off from awareness of a massive segment of the self. Massive dissociative reactions are, thus, a primitive means of dealing with rising anxiety.

The symptoms of dissociative disorder are both psychological and psychophysiological since, according to West (1967), the dissociated person's behavior reflects a compromise reached by the psyche and the central nervous system in an effort to manage the information being pressed upon them from the outside world. Essentially, an "information overload" occurs—the mind boggles at the input forced on it by the outside world and some parts of this awareness are cast out of consciousness.

When our sensory apparatus is disturbed by drugs, fatigue, loss of sleep, or artificially induced sensory deprivation, there is a related disruption of consciousness. Even the "hypnotism of the road" (when drivers seem transfixed by the road's dividing line and suffer decreased sensitivity to stimuli vital to safe driving) is a kind of simple alteration of consciousness that can have fatal consequences for life and limb. Unfortunately, the neurophysiology of psychoneurotic dissociative reactions remains a theoretical, speculative, and neglected area of study.

Dissociative reactions can, however, easily be produced experimentally using hypnosis as a tool. The altered state of consciousness attendant on the hypnotic trance is, of course, an artificial state incapable of being reproduced exactly in real life. But it can serve as an exceptional demonstration of the bare, finger-tip grip most of us have on consciousness and personal identity. The hypnotized person can be instructed to behave as if he were someone other than himself, as if he valued other than the standards he has lived by, and he manages this extremely well with little prompting.

In much the same fashion, the normal condition of the human psyche can be altered most simply by eliminating the casual sensory input (sights, smells, sounds, feelings, etc.) that fill the life of all of us. Floating suspended in a tank of water kept at body temperature, nose-plugged to eliminate odors, eyes covered to reduce visual stimulation, and ears bombarded by steady a-tonal sound, man's fragile self can no longer apprehend the world in the usual ways. Our grasp of reality can only be described as tenuous—a condition that can exist in a stable fashion only under quite restrictive circumstances. This observation suggests that our proper task might better be to account for how the parts of the self remain integrated rather than how they become dissociated from one another.

A number of the hallucinogenic drugs—LSD, peyote, or mescaline—can chemically manufacture a state of consciousness in which time, place, and identity get scrambled in ways that resemble purely clinical dissociation. Fatigue can produce a similar effect. Going without sleep for an extended period of time loosens the grasp of reality. Hallucinations, delusions, a sense of alienation, depersonalization, or dissociation from the real world are common denominators to a variety of sensory experiences.

The most usual symptomatic forms of dissociative reactions are amnesia, somnambulism, fugue states, and multiple personality. With

amnesia, memory is "lost" for a period of time usually following some
psychologically traumatic event. The memory loss most often involves an
absence of the ability to recollect one's personal identity: Who am I?
Somnambulism, in contrast, is a much more common experience. Somnambulism, or sleepwalking, usually appears in childhood but may occur
at any time that the problems of living become particularly stressful.
Fugue states occur when the person loses all sense of identity, abandons
his normal environment, and may establish a new life and identity for
himself. [In the dissociative reaction labeled multiple personality we have
a dramatic demonstration of the possibility of autonomous, independent
existence of distinct personalities in the same person.]

The Dynamics of Dissociation

Each of us has experienced at least a mild form of dissociative reaction.
There are times for all of us when persons, places, and events seem somehow removed from immediacy and become distant, strange, or alien.
These modest feelings of oddness, distance, detachment, or estrangement
occur as a consequence of distressing personal tension or threat. We are
dazed by incomprehensible events (the death of a loved one, the assas-
sination of an admired leader, or a downturn in our personal affairs) and
preoccupied with working through our problems. We do not appear to
be "ourselves" to others but, in time, we shake loose from our worries,
anxieties, and personal difficulties and become our old selves.

That temporary dissociative reactions occur should come as no sur-
prise. Each of us is, psychologically, an active battlefield of warring
tendencies, conflicting impulses, competing urges, and incompatible
wishes. We lose our bearings when confronted with complicated social
dilemmas and display what can best be described as a transient coping
pathology when exposed to severe personal pressure. For some this becomes an all-consuming way of life in which dissociation of one facet of
the self from its related aspects is an immediate, predictable, and dominant feature of psychological response to the threat of anxiety.

Dissociative reactions are described as abnormal when such experiences become exceptionally intense, are beyond one's capacity to control
them, or last beyond modest lengths of time. At a moderate level of
intensity, there is simple isolation from a painful situation. When this dissociation becomes more severe, there is a steady progression from depersonalization and estrangement, through fantasy or dreamlike states.

The dissociative response to anxiety is "chosen" or "selected" unconsciously to meet the pressing demands of an emergent, anxiety-provoking
situation. In a person whose psychological resources are varied and

sophisticated, a more complex and less damaging management of anxiety might be forthcoming; the individual for whom only psychic dissociation will provide adequate protection from anxiety is adjusting as best he can to problems with which he cannot cope in any other way.

The fragmenting of the self in response to threat is accomplished by repressive devices that are more thorough-going than usual in the neuroses —a repression so extensive that it dominates the symptom picture. In psychoanalytic theory, the sexual impulses are the most likely candidates for massive repression. Sexuality, and conflict about sexual impulses, occupy a central, but not exclusive, position in dissociative reactions.

The defensive formula of those psychoneuroses marked by dissociative features is fairly straightforward. The forbidden and anxiety-provoking impulses that were dealt with originally by simple repression break into consciousness despite defensive attempts to remove them from consciousness. Repression, having failed, makes necessary a next, more severe step to protect the psychological integrity of the person. Entire experiences, persons, and events are relegated to unconsciousness and a vital part of one's whole self simply ceases to exist.

Unfortunately, this separation of self into distinct parts is less than perfect. In what is called a fugue state, for example, the impulse rendered unconscious may still be expressed during a brief interruption in the conscious state. Such symbolic expressions of the forbidden impulse may, as an illustration, occur in periods of somnambulism when sleep has altered the watchfulness usually exercised over one's conscious life. Repression that is so extensive is a primitive defensive move since it cuts off the possibility of dealing with anxiety-provoking psychological issues in a more mature fashion. The separation of one part of the self from other segments of personality inevitably pauperizes the ego and limits its user to less than sophisticated patterns of relating to others.

Let us now look in greater detail at the forms and varieties of dissociation that can occur in human beings beginning with the most common of such experiences—sleepwalking.

Sleepwalking

We all dream and, in dreams, we may express in fantasy the impulses, conflicts, and concerns we withheld from consciousness during our waking hours. Asleep and dreaming we are dissociated from the limitations and restraints of reality—anything is possible in the dream world. In addition, the watchful alertness of the ego and super ego are diminished in this semiconscious state and forbidden impulses and urges are loosed to play in the mind. When these dream fantasies are sufficiently vivid and compelling, we may rise from the bed and act out solutions to the conflicts or physically express some part of our forbidden wishes or urges.

This "normal" form of psychoneurosis tells us something about the state of the individual's psychological well-being. The sleepwalker can rarely recall the events that transpire in this state of dissociation, and this memory loss is similar in many respects to the full-blown amnesias of persons with more severe emotional disorders. Somnambulism most often occurs in adolescence and reflects the turmoil of shedding childhood and assuming an adult form, but it is not always an isolated symptom. Sandler (1945) reported that in 22 instances of reported somnambulism in the armed forces, 18 of the sleepwalkers had been referred for psychiatric treatment for other symptoms.

Amnesia and the Fugue States

The dissociative reaction of amnesia is not limited to the psychoneuroses. It can occur suddenly (as a consequence of brain damage attendant on accident or injury) or slowly (in the degeneration of the brain with increasing age). These cases reflect a physiological rather than psychogenic loss of the ability to register, retain, or recall the who, what, why, when, and where of life.

In psychoneurotic dissociation, important facts and information are retained but, for purely psychological reasons, unavailable to consciousness. In the true amnesias of a psychogenic variety, for example, the principal loss is that of identity. The individual continues to make his way through life and maintains his previous patterns of habit, belief, attitude, and response but these are disconnected from the painful persons, places, and situations of the past.

The amnesia victim is rarely a paragon of maturity or stable adjustment. He has been described, rather, as suggestible, dependent, immature, and egocentric. He is psychologically unable to cope successfully with life during ordinary times and takes psychic flight when troubles beset him. The "new" personality the amnesiac assumes could hardly be expected to be more mature than the one just abandoned; it is rather a loose conglomeration of bits and pieces of the old wedded uncomfortably with new attempts to find a more workable formula for living.

When an altered state of consciousness is used to escape from an oppressive situation, it is described as a fugue state. In an amnesia *without* fugue the patient may wander aimlessly while confused about who he is, what he is doing, and where he belongs. As he becomes aware that things are not as they ought to be, he may seek help to discover his identity.

When amnesia obliterates an intolerable set of life circumstances it frees its victim to establish a new and different identity and, optimistically, begin a new life in which he will fare better. He moves away from his previous ties and into a new set of social and personal arrangements in a state of split-consciousness in which revealing memories of the past must be distorted or kept completely from consciousness. Some of the most dramatic tabloid accounts of combined amnesia and fugue have been those in which the victim is discovered, years later, leading a new and, often, bigamous life. Males who bear the responsibility of working and supporting a family are most often the ones who run when the pressure of life overcomes them.

The case of Mac K. can be used to illustrate the logic of amnesia as a means of retreat from the trials and tribulations of life.

MAC K.

In combination, Mac's resentment of his position in life and his feeling that he deserved much better, his predilection for ignoring unpleasant reality, the harassment he felt he was suffering in life, and his proclivity for losing himself in the personality of make-believe characters all added up to a readiness to run away from life by dumping his former self and beginning all over again. He had practiced running and hiding throughout his life and had simply become more and more adept at getting out from under when the pressure mounted beyond his capacity to manage it.

This time in Mac's life proved to be the culmination of a series of events, and he assembled, through amnesia, a final and complete portrait of a man whose psyche plays tricks on him when these tricks make him feel less pain. A part of Mac's consciousness separated from the whole of his awareness and he actually became two persons. One Mac K. had memories that included a wife, children, a job, friends, and a mounting pile of troubles. The other Mac K. had all the recollections of self except those that would remind him that he had failed in some important way to become what he thought he ought to become. Mac No. 1 had been unable to achieve what he ought to and was reminded of it at every turn. He was a man beset by difficulties, shortcomings, limitations, and awareness of failure. Mac No. 2 was a new man reborn without recollection of hurdles never mastered or tasks sloppily and only partly accomplished. He was still young enough to run more successfully the same race he felt he had lost before, and he was a man unencumbered by responsibility that would limit his capacity to exercise his talents. He could play-act, for example, without returning to home and family. In his new life he could, with clear conscience, idle away the hours of morning discussing with great seriousness the fine points of technique with novice actors who hung avidly on his every word. With his flair for fantasy Mac had little difficulty filling the missing years with romantic deceptions and half-truths that described his life as he wished it to be rather than as it really had been. The gap in his existence could be decorated with events and happenings that would make his person more attractive, mysterious, and romantic than it really was.

What happened to Mac was an extreme version of what is a part of all of us in miniature. With Mac it achieved proportions beyond what most of us could manage comfortably. Mac did what many of us do in fantasy but few in real life. Mac K., however, had adopted a solution to his problem that was destined to fail, primarily because Mac was only partly ready to drop his past for an unknown and shaky future; he was uncomfortable with the solution that he had chosen, but it was this or nothing at all for him (McNeil, 1967; pp. 41–42).

Multiple Personality

The amnesiac who has shed one life and undertaken another presents a quite dramatic instance of the dissociative process sustained over a period of weeks, months, or years. For a rare few, dissociative reactions occur early in life, distort personality development in its formative years, and produce an adult whose psychic structure houses more than one distinct personality.

A normal counterpart of multiple personality can be seen in persons whose style of life differs starkly in different situations or at different moments in time. Seemingly circumspect, moral persons who lead secret lives of corruption and immorality do not really fit the definition of dissociation if they are aware of these discrepancies between the two sets of behavior and simply find it wise socially to present only the most acceptable facade to public view. By the same token those whose moods vacillate rapidly and unpredictably day by day do not fit the criteria of multiple personality since such mood swings can most often be accounted for in a variety of other more parsimonious ways.

It is when more than one organized personality exists independently in the same person and these separate selves are dissociated one from another that the diagnosis of multiple personality is rightfully made.

When such separate personalities exist, they seldom are reported to be equally stable, mature, or well-organized entities. One pattern of personality organization is usually dominant, but this may alternate on occasion with the submissive other part of the self. The dominant personality may be unaware of the existence of its submissive counterpart (Thigpen and Cleckley, 1957). According to West (1967), some dissociative states do take on a frenzied or violent form. In these instances acute dissociative reactions appear quite suddenly and last for just a brief period of time but during these episodes (for which the patient usually has amnesia), he may run berserk and violently attack everyone in his path. This dissociative reaction is usually in response to an accumulation of frustrations so intense that violence and frenzy may seem to be the only way of relieving tension.

What can produce such a bizarre distortion of human consciousness? At a minimum, it must take a unique combination of traumatic or stressful experiences early in life and these must be dealt with by reliance on the mechanisms of denial and massive repression as exclusive ways of relieving pressure. It takes a sense of estrangement, depersonalization, and experience with mild dissociative reactions over a period of years to culminate in the dramatic splitting-off of consciousness reflected by multiple personality. The longer the process has been underway, the more distinct and separate the various personalities can come to be; the longer these particular mechanisms are used exclusively to deal with problems, the easier it becomes to fall into a pattern of "dropping out" parts of conscious experience.

SUMMARY

The need to avoid the painful and frightening experience of severe anxiety can trigger a series of psychic maneuvers that produce behavior we call neurotic. While there is much we should realistically be anxious about in daily life, most of our anxieties are acquired as we learn the complicated series of rules and expectations society holds out for each of us. Neurotic anxiety reactions are occasioned by the failure of repression effectively to remove forbidden or personally unacceptable impulses from conscious awareness. Faced with unbearable anxiety, the individual defends himself. Two examples of symptom patterns produced by defense mechanisms are phobic reactions and dissociative reactions.

In phobic reactions, anxiety is warded off by denying its connection to the impulse being defended against and attaching it to some other object, person, or situation in the external environment. These, then, can be avoided and the person is anxiety-free as long as he is not forced to confront the dreaded effect of his phobia. This fairly simple and direct psychic compromise appears most often among children ("the neurosis of childhood") since much of the real world is frightening to them or beyond their capacity to manage. Traditional one-to-one psychotherapeutic methods have long been applied to phobic sufferers and, recently, behavioral therapists have succeeded in relieving such extreme fears using conditioning and desensitization techniques.

Dissociative reactions represent a different, and more severe, means of dealing with anxiety. The average person has only a tenuous hold on consciousness, i.e., his capacity to integrate and analyze sensations and perceptions can easily be disordered by drugs, fatigue, or severe social pressure. The mild feelings of strangeness, depersonalization, and disconnection from the world that all of us experience from time to time are dissociative reactions that, when intense, can produce sleepwalking, amnesia, a fugue-like flight from reality, or the development of multiple personalities within a single psychic structure. The ego can fragment into distinct parts and destroy the integrity of the conscious self.

Obsessive-Compulsive Reactions 3

Many of the so-called witches of the 15th century revealed to the inquisitors of that era symptoms that, today, would be classified as obsessive-compulsive in nature. When the obsessive urge to stick out one's tongue while passing a church was compulsively acted out, the merging of inescapable idea and irresistible action were ascribed to the influence of the devil. Nemiah (1967) observed that by the 19th century, "the explanation of the phenomena has been shifted from external supernatural forces to a consideration of the inner workings of the human mind. Demonology has been replaced by psychology—a natural science" (p. 920).

The first 20th century theories attributed obsessive-compulsive reactions to a diminution of mental energy. This "weakness" resulted in disorganization of the mental functions and a scrambling of "the forces of *will* and *attention* that ordinarily allowed each of us to perceive himself and his environment *realistically,* and to perform actions appropriate to that correctly perceived reality" (Nemiah, 1967; p. 920). Thus a kind of mental anarchy was thought to exist in which powerful emotions force us to entertain alien thoughts and to perform actions objectionable to ourselves and others. This explanation of obsessive-compulsive reactions was quite mechanical, i.e., it predicted such a pattern of behavior for all persons suffering a diminution of mental energy. It was unaware of unconscious processes in man. The early theorists failed to understand that those strange ideas and unusual actions were not alien at all—they were, rather, unrecognized, unconscious internal promptings ineffectively denied access to consciousness.

Freud supplied the missing theoretical link and tied it closely to the course of early childhood development. Freud suggested that obsessive-compulsive reactions were psychodynamic rather than demonological in nature and that they were responses rooted in the early experience of the child. Today, the obsessive-compulsive reactions are of interest primarily to those of psychoanalytic persuasion. In 1966, for example, several issues of the *International Journal of Psycho-Analysis* were devoted to a reexamination of the orthodox views of this disorder.

Obsessive-compulsive disorders make up approximately 12 percent of the neurotic disturbances (Laughlin, 1967). The deterioration of obsession into severe depression is a common complication, although the risk of suicide, alcoholism, or drug addiction is less than usual (Rosenberg, 1968). Some theoreticians have suggested more firstborn or only children are subject to this kind of personality disorganization (Kayton and Borge, 1967) as a consequence of exclusive exposure to adults during childhood (without the relief provided by siblings) and the higher expectations for achievement set for them by parents.

THE COMPONENTS OF OBSESSIVE-COMPULSIVE REACTIONS

Since so many persons who consider themselves "normal" are subject to moderate obsessive-compulsive reactions from time to time, a true appraisal of the frequency of this disorder is hard to achieve. Obsessive-compulsive reactions are shaped over a life time for most persons and unmistakable evidence of this problem is usually visible early in life for both men and women.

A Case of Obsession-Compulsion

The case of Georgia M. will illustrate the degree to which obsessive-compulsive reactions may dominate the whole of an individual's existence and convert positive relationships with others into negative reactions.

First, the description of obsession by the victim:

> I can't get to sleep unless I am sure everything in the house is in its proper place so that when I get up in the morning the house is organized. I work like mad to set everything straight before I go to bed, but, when I get up in the morning, I can think of a thousand things that I ought to do. I know some of the things are ridiculous, but I feel better if I get them done, and I can't stand to know something needs doing and I

Coleman stresses the importance to the obsessive of organizing a secure and predictable life in the face of a world that is hopelessly disordered, threatening, untidy, and unpredictable. If the world is a dangerous place, then at least one corner of it is made stable, reliable, programmed, and safe. The librarians of the world have been stereotyped as obsessive-compulsive personalities who fall back on a system, order, and regularity both to reduce the external threat of disorder and to deny the reality of impulses that threaten to invert the style of life they have so carefully cultivated. Unfortunately, ritual and order are poor substitutes for feeling and spontaneity in life. The rigidity of obsessive behavior shuts the door to new experience.

The Obsessive-Compulsive Style

David Shapiro (1965) suggests that if we look beyond the anxiety and the impulses being defended against in obsessive disorder we can see some characteristic patterns of psychological make-up that are essential to our understanding of the person and his neurotic style of life. He notes, for example, that obsessive-compulsive persons take a rigid approach to action and reaction in life. This rigidity may take the form of persisting in the pursuit of a course of action that is absurd, a stiff, formal social comportment, or a dogmatic and opinionated style of thinking. Some types of obsessive personalities may be exceptionally alert and attentive; yet their ability to concentrate may be focused so intently on fine detail that they cannot apprehend the larger situation and thus fail to respond properly to it, e.g., they may lose track of the plot of a movie because they are so immersed in commenting on the film's technical flaws.

In addition, Shapiro suggests that this cognitive rigidity is complemented by unusual involvement in activity. The obsessive may be a busy person, but his activity is not quite an effortless engagement in a variety of interests and tasks. It is, rather, a strain-laden, driven, "being trapped" in work whether it interests the victim or not. The deadline set for completion of each and every task may become a fixed, rigid, absolute dictum for the obsessive that he frets about, and he suffers disappointment and anger when it is not met. Once he becomes caught up in a task (feeling he "should" do it), he is no longer free to stop or to do less than a perfect job. He imposes standards and moral imperatives on himself and these compel him to labor mightily on each and every assignment that comes his way. The obsessive could never subscribe to a philosophy that says "only some jobs worth doing are worth doing well."

The obsessive attraction to work and the compulsive total immersion in a task indicate that it would be difficult for such persons to enjoy the rest and relaxation of vacations. Vacations would be perceived as "absence from work" and would be as meticulously organized and fussed over as any other serious assignment. They would not fulfill the prescription for a regressive escape from responsibility most of us call vacations. An obsessive-compulsive personality must feel uncomfortable when exposed to temptation to abandon his style of life. As Shapiro (1965) indicates, pleasure for its own sake is, for the obsessive, likened to losing control over one's life.

The indecisiveness of obsessive-compulsive persons is also legendary. When every possible factor and force has finally been carefully measured and weighed and a decision seems imminent, some new fact, possibility, or probability occurs to the obsessed person and the decision-making process grinds to a halt. In this manner he engages in psychological acrobatics to avoid becoming the source of a decision that might later prove to be in error. If a decision *must* be made, the obsessed person is happiest when he can invoke a policy, rule, or logical principle to relieve him of responsibility for the conclusion finally reached. The physical and psychological effort—the sheer energy expended in the decision-making process—is enormous. Most of us "worry" now and then (rather, we ruminate excessively and fruitlessly examine and re-examine the same set of facts), but "worry" is not an integral part of our whole style of life.

Finally, Shapiro describes a characteristic "loss of reality" in which obsessive-compulsive persons become concerned and worried about a variety of possible, if not probable, events. Often these concerns are located in the nebulous area of health and physical well-being. This is not full-blown delusion, however, since the obsessed person is concerned with the probability of illness more than the truth of being diseased.

The important observation, for Shapiro, is that the obsessive-compulsive person displays a style of life that seems to reach beyond the minimal requisites of dealing with anxiety, impulse, and defense; that there is a style as well as content to obsession. Certainly it is fair to say that living with one's symptoms has a different flair after it has been practiced over a lifetime.

Obsessive-Compulsive Defenses

Freud described the defense mechanisms used by the obsessive-compulsive to ward off anxiety as isolation, undoing, and reaction formation.

1. Isolation

The thoughts of most of us contain both an idea and our emotions or feelings about the idea. When these two aspects of thought are separated (the emotion dissociated from the thought) we have the experience of the obsessed person, i.e., there may be an objectionable thought but the emotion that would usually accompany it is absent. Thus, the obsessed person may be plagued by the fantasy that all the members of his family are dead or horribly mutilated. He is fully aware of these thoughts but reacts to them in a neutral (nonemotional) fashion since the full and true meaning of his thoughts is hidden from him. If he were to become aware that his fantasy of the dead and mutilated bodies of his loved ones were accurate reflections of his own unadmitted urges and wishes, he would be flooded with guilt-laden emotions that might destroy him. As it is, he is mystified by the unwelcome intrusion of such images into his thoughts and, mildly annoyed, seeks unsuccessfully to rid himself of them. Since he has isolated the thought from its usual emotion, he is disturbed but not in panic over its appearance. The defense mechanism of isolation has protected him against the destructive impact of a full awareness of the contents of his psychic life.

2. Undoing

When isolation proves to be an inadequate defense against anxiety, a new maneuver is called for to undo or cancel out the hostile and forbidden impulses. The obsessed person tries to undo or correct the fancied wrongs he may have inadvertently committed and denies access to consciousness of the forbidden impulse by checking and rechecking to be certain he has not acted in an incorrect manner.

In a classic form of this defensive behavior, a person suffering from the nagging fear that he has accidentally killed all the members of his family by leaving the kitchen gas jets turned on, reassures himself by checking, rechecking, and checking again to be sure the gas jets are fully off. The problem with actions designed to undo is that each such action is a stimulus that triggers again the obsessive thought the person needs so much to deny. Thus, he is caught in a vicious circle of action-reaction-action. Each action relieves anxiety at the same moment that it stimulates it anew—this cycle need never begin if the defense of isolation is adequate to the task.

3. Reaction Formation

Reaction formation (doing the opposite of the repressed wish or impulse) is a defense that has as its aim a longer range goal of organizing fairly permanent character traits rather than simply defending against the anxiety provoked by each new impulse breakthrough. Behavior based on reaction formation may appear to others as exaggerated and sometimes inappropriate, but it provides a kind of permanent protection from the anxiety that the defenses of isolation and undoing seem unable to achieve. The lives of some persons are systematically organized, "like clock-work," to assure a dependable, predictable world in which they are protected against their own unwelcome impulse to kick over the traces, abandon responsibility, and seek pleasure rather than approval of others.

For some persons, excessive cleanliness, kindness, and concern for others may mask the urge to express the opposite of these patterns of behavior—to soil, be self-seeking, and injure others. If the feared and denied impulse is intense, the degree of reaction formation may need to be equally intense. Thus, the impulse to be cruel to others may be denied by an obsessive kindness that is so extensive it renders the individual incapable of being unkind even when such behavior might be appropriate (e.g., when it is vital to a child's safety to restrict rather than indulge him).

Obsessive Doubt

Life is full of natural uncertainties that are a prime source of question and doubt for all of us. At the moment these questions and doubts are finally resolved they seem to be replaced by new, more puzzling ones. The obsessive-compulsive person may display a grossly exaggerated, paralyzing doubt about both the vital questions of life as well as the trivia of existence. In some instances the deep doubt that surrounds fundamental questions of life (to soil or to be clean, to hate or to love) gets displaced by the trivia or technicalities of existence since, at least, the minutia of day by day living can be dealt with effectively even if life's bigger issues are unsolvable. The intensity with which an individual searches for an answer to the meaning of life may reflect more his indecision about expressing or not expressing his basic impulses than philosophic concern with life's mysteries.

The future is, for all of us, a "probabalistic" set of events and most of us hesitate to make commitments about the unknown.. The obsessive personality, however, not only fears the future but is irresolute about past action. He not only worries about what will be, he is uncertain of the correctness of those actions he has taken in the past; he fears his memory deceives him and he is made anxious both by errors he may have committed as well as errors that might be made in the future.

Ritual and Compulsion

Compulsive actions are designed to avoid anxiety, but when anxiety sits constantly outside the conscious doorway such actions may become ritualized and require constant repetition to assure one's psychic safety. The victim feels *obliged* to count, touch, wash his hands, check environmental conditions, or repeat behavior patterns even if these actions seem absurd and meaningless. The comfort and relief such actions provide are sufficient justification for the behavior—it just feels better if the ritual is performed and it feels miserable if it is omitted.

The exactness of the ritual—every move is made precisely as it was in the past—has a magical quality about it which tells us the victim of the compulsion is reassuring himself by nullifying the possibility that a forbidden impulse has accidentally loosened its bonds and found a way to destructive, anxiety-provoking expression. In Kolb's (1968) words ". . . the defensive patterns of the compulsions resemble penance, atonement, and punishments, or serve as precautions, prohibitions, and restrictions. In many ways, they are closely allied psychologically to the ceremonies and taboos that primitive people devise as protections against demonological and other supernatural forces" (p. 485).

Hypnosis lets us glimpse something of the inner workings of compulsive, ritualistic behavior. When an individual is hypnotized and a suggestion implanted—e.g., when you receive a phone call during which the code word Napoleon is spoken, you will be compelled to come to my house bearing one card from the deck, the Ace of Spades—the hypnotized person finds himself compelled to carry out this senseless, irrational action. He knows his behavior is bizarre and unreasonable and he tries to resist with all the will-power he can command. But, resisting the stupid impulse produces a wave of anxiety. So, despite his embarrassment, he carries the ridiculous action to its conclusion.

Nonsense rituals induced by hypnosis are a fair counterpart to the need for ritualistic behavior that is common to obsessive-compulsive reactions. The obsessive thought intrudes itself into consciousness uninvited; the action becomes necessary to avoid the onslaught of anxiety. The neurotic individual is trapped in a pattern of his own defensive making; he must act as he does or suffer anxiety. He decides, rather, to act out those rituals that make him comfortable and to live with their senselessness.

Obsession and Depression

Cameron (1963) notes that a symptom pattern of neurotic depression rather than obsessive-compulsive reaction is simply the substitution of one kind of guilt neurosis for another. In both instances a prime source of conflict is between what is and what ought to be—between conscience and reality. While obsessive-compulsive persons tie up energy in an active "doing" to escape anxiety, the neurotic depressive "gives up," demeans himself, denigrates his capacities and abilities, becomes helpless, and throws himself on the mercy of those closest to him (Benda, 1967). The independence and self-assertiveness of the obsessive makes him seem incapable of accepting help in changing his style of life, but behind the facade of unworthiness of the depressive lies a more formidable barrier to accepting help—hostility and resentment about being forced to abandon the self totally to the care of others.

While some who suffer obsessive-compulsive reactions seek traditional psychotherapeutic assistance, this symptom pattern proves to be refractory to treatment. As we might expect, the earlier treatment begins, the greater the likelihood of altering his style of life. The more rigid the system of thought and action becomes, the less likely it is to be abandoned by the patient.

Psychotherapeutic treatment of obsessive disorder, with or without depressive overtones, is a particularly difficult task. In exceptionally severe cases in which hospitalization and home confinement are required, treatment of the obsessive poses unique problems since penetration of the patient's total absorption with obsessive thoughts and compulsive actions is difficult to achieve. Recently, attempts have been made to use a conditioned inhibition approach to treatment in which the patient is placed in a light hypnotic trance, told to "act out" his obsessions, and then given electroconvulsive shock. In Rubin's (1967) report of treatment of four patients (who had previously failed to respond to psychiatric treatment), all were said to recover immediately. It will require substantial additional evidence to be certain a new and productive approach to treatment has been uncovered, but the limited success of traditional methods has given some urgency to the search for a new means of treatment.

SUMMARY

The invasion of the mind by unsummoned, repulsive, or objectionable thoughts coupled with an intensive urge to engage in impulsive actions describe the obsessive-compulsive reaction. Such patterns of behavior are a modest part of the life of each of us as we organize, systematize, and sometimes ritualize our work, our play, and our daily existence. When we are anxious we seek order to reassure ourselves that we can control our environment and thus our lives.

The obsessive-compulsive person develops a defensive style of life that is stiff, formal, rigid, and oriented oppressively to work. The defense mechanisms regularly used to ward off anxiety are isolation (separating the emotion from the intrusive thought), undoing (behaving in a way to be certain forbidden impulses were not acted on), and reaction formation (doing the opposite of the repressed wish or impulse). Despite these defensive attempts to escape anxiety, the life of the obsessive is filled with doubt, ritual, and compulsion. The obsessive-compulsive reaction is costly to the way of life of its victim.

Depressive Reaction 4

The mood disorder labeled neurotic depression produces an unmistakable clinical picture that differs from psychotic depression most obviously in the degree of apathetic retardation of all bodily and psychological functions and less obviously in the amount of dependence on others and severity of regression to an earlier, dependent state (Mendelson, 1967). This, then, is a unitary theoretical concept that views all depressions as similar in kind but distinguishable in degree. Implicit in this description is the view that neurotic depression is a modest response to modest pressures just as the psychotic depressive reaction is a response to severe pressures with an equally disruptive and destructive psychological disturbance. As Beck (1967) indicates, neurotic depression is most often a reaction to clearly defined, stressful, external situations which, for most of us, can be alleviated by a change in life circumstances or an alteration of interpersonal relationships.

Bonime (1966) states, "Depression is a way of living—a sick way" (p. 239). It is a psychological condition marked by "an exaggeratedly lowered mood precipitated by a definable loss, frustration, or disappointment. The patient shows diminution of incentive, retardation of activity, a decline in enjoyment or anticipation of his customary physical, social, affective, or intellectual sources of pleasure. He tends toward a sense of helplessness, hopelessness, and inconsolability. . . . His mental processes remain intact, though tending to manifest mild or moderate degrees of sluggishness, which he may tentatively overcome by effort. . . . In addition to feeling excessively the weight of responsibility, the patient may be frustrated, angered, even made anxious, by an unaccustomed

disorganization, lack of persistence, and scatter in his approach to tasks"
(Bonime, 1966; p. 241).

THE DYNAMICS OF DEPRESSION

As Buss (1966) indicates, ". . . neurotic depression may be viewed as
a reaction to failure or loss: failure to solve important life problems,
failure to cope with conflict, or loss of an important relationship" (p. 61).
He notes that the symptoms of hysteria or obsessive-compulsive neurosis
represent circumscribed and clear attempts to avoid or escape from
anxiety while the symptoms of depression are a kind of vague, diffuse
surrender to the difficulties of life. The depressed person is disturbed
emotionally (affectively) by apathy, pessimism, and melancholy and his
motor (muscular) apparatus is slowed down and rendered useless.

Dynamically, the neurotic depressive is victimized by regression to
earlier phases of development and must once again deal with the unresolved conflicts and problems of a bygone age—he responds as a child
to adult problems. He becomes a helpless person dependent on the care
and security he forces others to provide for him. He proclaims his
culpability, throws himself on the mercy of more powerful persons in
his environment, and frees himself of responsibility. When normal depression occurs—as it will for anyone whose frustration tolerance is
exceeded—the loss in self-esteem and the unhappy mood are temporary.
In neurosis, the victim fails to recover his precarious balance; his ability
to compensate for external stress is no longer adequate to the task.

While a neurotic depression can appear suddenly and unexpectedly,
it most often is a reaction to tension and anxiety that accumulate as a
result of a series of minor crises piled one atop another. Threat, frustration, loss, or new responsibilities and obligations tip the psychic scales,
and the mounting difficulties in living trigger a full-blown depression.
Bodily complaints increase in number and severity and a characteristic
confusion, inability to concentrate, waning of interest in the outside
world, and self-deprecation come to the fore. The hatred the depressive
unconsciously feels for himself now dominates his life.

According to Cameron (1963), the regression of the neurotic depressive revives childhood conflicts about being loved, accepted, and wanted.
Anger and resentment over feelings of not being loved (or being an
unlovable person) are consciously denied even though they are unmistakably evident in the tone and content of the complaints the depressed individual lodges against the way the world is put together.

The probable dynamic basis for neurotically depressed behavior suggests, first, that such persons have deep oral needs that are not adequately gratified in daily life. The basic trust of others and confidence in the self that should develop in infancy and childhood seem to be absent for neurotics who get depressed. They seem to remain fixated on unresolved personal and interpersonal conflicts about dependence-independence and lovability-unlovability. It is possible for a child to grow to adulthood presenting a facade of self-confidence and self-acceptance to himself and others only to have this appearance eroded by successive failures to accomplish what others expect of him and what he demands of himself.

DEPRESSION AND SUICIDE

Suicide is the tenth major cause of death in the United States since, each year, more than 20,000 of our fellow citizens take their own life. By every evaluation we can make, this is a highly conservative estimate. According to Hendin (1967), "The average yearly United States suicide rate of 10.5 per 100,000 places this country in the middle of any international scale. Ireland, Chile, and New Zealand, for example, consistently have suicide rates below 6 per 100,000; Japan, Denmark, Sweden, Austria, West Germany, and Hungary have suicide rates averaging 20 per 100,000" (p. 1170).

Yet, the extensive bibliographies on suicide compiled by Farberow and Schneidman (1961) and Resnik (1968) suggest that professional concern with the act of suicide is probably out of proportion to the actual number of those who take their own lives.

Suicide, according to Weiss (1966), involves three vital etiological factors, "the group attitudes in each particular society, the adverse extraneous situations that the person must meet, and the interaction of these with his character and personality" (p. 115). It is important to note that each of us reacts to adversity in an individualistic way, yet there have been societies in which suicide is unknown or its rate extremely low. In addition, it is difficult to assess the frequency of all kinds of suicide. The depressed person who threatens to end his life, finally does so, and leaves a suicide note explaining the reasons for this action presents what is apparently the clearest case. Less obvious are the cases of the multitude of persons who neglect their health and well being, have fatal accidents, or provoke assaults by others. This group (Farberow and Schneidman, 1961) may by far outnumber those who destroy themselves in an unmistakably calculated and deliberate fashion.

Thus, the seriously depressed person is a source of anxiety to others not only because of the acute suffering and despair he expresses but because of the possibility that he may terminate his own life. As Alex Pokorny (1968) notes, most of what we know of suicide and the depressive condition is riddled with fallacies, old wive's tales, and superstition. Among these myths about suicide, he lays to rest the notion that "people who talk about suicide won't commit suicide." A great many careful studies report that nearly three-fourths of those who actually carry the act to completion have alluded to the possibility in advance. With the percentage so high, it is apparent that those who threaten to end their lives may, sooner or later, succeed in achieving their goal—their suicide rate is 35 times that of the general population. Pokorny also observes that suicide seldom occurs without advance warning and this warning is most often in the form of a direct statement of intent to do away with one's self.

Pokorny reports that those who commit suicide and those who attempt suicide must be viewed as overlapping but distinct populations. Many attempt suicide but do not succeed; their lack of success is not the same as a "failure," i.e., the dramatic attempt at suicide is often used as a signal that interpersonal relationships are disturbed and help is needed. Often just the gesture of trying to take one's life is sufficient to evoke the needed sympathetic response from loved ones.

There has been an *absolute* increase in the number of persons who kill themselves each year but there is little *relative* increase in rate of suicide in proportion to the population. This relative rate shifts over time (low in wartime; high during economic depression) in response to major cultural changes. In combination, personal and social forces produce depression in individuals and this psychological state naturally entertains thoughts of escape by ending physical existence.

Suppose we view suicide as an extreme expression of the depressives' urge to be punished for the "failure and worthlessness" they feel is their lot. Self-punishment is called for since few of us treat depressives as badly as they feel they deserve.

There are a number of theoretical explanations of why an individual comes to attack himself rather than others. A purely profit-and-loss approach to the consequences of turning aggressive impulses against the self would have to entertain a number of possibilities such as the following:

1. If we can accept the premise that it is possible for a person, while learning to manage his aggressive impulses, to introject or incorporate some symbolic representation of the punishing parent into his psychic economy, then we can understand that one "gain"

from self-punitive action would be to punish not the self but the "other" inside him. In this way a symbolic revenge might be taking place. This is not a theory that is easily judged in terms of its face validity, since it relies heavily on unconscious events—events not available for conscious inspection.

2. Self-punishment also serves to ward off the punishment that one might anticipate would come from others. An aggressive act which would normally bring retaliation from the injured victim can go without punishment if the offended party feels the aggressor has "suffered enough at his own hand." Being one's own jury and executioner has the additional advantage of increasing the chance that punishment will not be excessive. Retaliation by those aggressed against may, in the heat of rage, exact a greater toll than self-punishment.

3. Self-punishment can be an expression of self-mastery at the same time that it assuages guilt. This is especially apparent in young children who will slap their own wrists for misbehavior but launch a vigorous protest if the parent attempts to inflict punishment. This tends to be a special case of conflict between the need for punishment and the continued effort to exert control over others in the environment. It has all the peculiar characteristics of the man who voluntarily walks the plank when his captors really offer him no alternative. It is an expression of independence even in the face of death.

4. An important element in self-punishment may be a simple matter of the most economical resolution of psychological forces. Overwhelmed by intense feelings of rage, finding that the overt expression of this rage toward objects outside the self is not feasible, and being unable to choke down the hostile feelings, the angry person may have no recourse other than attacking himself or assaulting some neutral object. The violent need for expression, coupled with the elimination of all but one object of attack, may produce self-punishment as the only alternative.

5. Self-punishment may serve the purpose for which it was originally intended. Our society strives to build into its members an internal set of controls and punishments to take the place of parents, police, and other enforcers. Ideally, we wish to have one policeman, jury, and judge inside the psychic structure of each of our citizens so that internal regulation will take the place of external coercion. Self-punishment, then, may merely be an expression of a lesson too well learned.

6. One of the most fascinating theories about the possible mean-

ing of self-punishment has been described by Theodore Reik (1941) in his book on *Masochism in Modern Man*. In this theory, punishment can serve as a commodity for barter with the conscience, a means of purchasing the right to induge in the forbidden act once again. A self-imposed penance can even the score, psychologically, and allow the same impulse free rein when opportunity next presents itself. Thus it is possible for an employer, who secretly believes that no one knows how to work hard any more, to criticize his workers and push them to greater effort, yet avoid guilt for his actions through punishing himself by working harder than anyone else. This kind of hostility can be expressed freely day after day because it is bought and paid for in the coinage of self-suffering.

Each of these possibilities has a natural logic about it, but the motivation for self-punishment may not be adequate to account for an act as extreme as suicide.

The social, religious, and legal reactions to suicide have varied in time from acceptance as a natural event, to condemnation by the church, to definition of it as a criminal act, and, finally, to its description as a product of mental derangement. The use of suicide as a legal method of punishment is known to every schoolboy familiar with the execution of Socrates, and for some centuries the suicide of martyrdom was glorified for its dedication to a high order of principle. Legal sanctions for suicide were eventually abandoned, but custom was more resistant to change, and social approval of suicide as a means of restoring personal honor still exists. The evolution of the conception that taking one's own life was a criminal act provided, at one time, for legal suicide if it was for good and sufficient reason, such as sickness, grief, or extreme weariness of life. In time, suicide became a crime—a puzzling crime in which the aggressor and the object of aggression were united in one person. It was a crime of murder in some systems of law and only a felony for others. In those instances where suicide and murder were equated, a variety of punishments was executed against the self-murderer; his property might be confiscated, he might be denied an honorable burial, or he might be hanged for his crime. Through the ages, actual or symbolic attempts have been made to separate the murderer from his victim by dismembering the body of the suicide and by burying the offending hand in one place and the body in another. The complexity of this problem furnished the wherewithal for a great philosophical debate lasting for centuries. Today, only a few

vestiges remain of the primitive attempts to achieve social punishment for the murderer of the self. Today's sanctions against suicide
are primarily moral, and an attempt to kill one's self can be dealt
with by the authorities only if there is a fair presumption of
mental illness (McNeil, 1959; pp. 239–41).

Of the depressed persons in the world, only a few will end their lives.
Most of them will find a less violent means of seeking what they consider
to be well-deserved punishment. Yet, the frequency of the drama of
attempted or successful suicide among depressives makes this act of
reasonable concern to all of us. Each of us will suffer the loss of love
objects during our lifetime, but only a few of us will react to these
losses with unremitting depression (Sternbach, 1965). Grief, for most
of us, will serve to break the bond of affection with lost loved ones
and allow us to return to the world of continuing interpersonal relationships (Averill, 1968).

THE TREATMENT OF DEPRESSION

There has always been a high correlation between depression and death
by suicide (Silverman, 1968). While it is possible to detect suicidal
patients in advance of their attempt at self-injury (Stone and Shein,
1968), conventional psychotherapeutic efforts are not always adequate
to forestall the act of personal destruction. In almost all cases, warning
signs are evident well in advance but total watchfulness is not always
possible. Frequently, a state of "calm" and a "lifting" of depressive
symptoms immediately precedes the suicidal act. It is as if the patient,
having finally decided to do away with himself, finds his mood changes
markedly as he sees the way clear to solving his problem (Keith-Spiegel
and Spiegel, 1967). This state of readiness for suicide occurs most frequently among women, since they attempt to do away with themselves
more often, but produces fatal results primarily among males, since
they succeed in suicide attempts with greater frequency (Davis, 1967;
1968). Male suicides use more violent methods, fail to seek medical
help before they attempt suicide, and are less often diagnosed as depressed when they are seen professionally.

The treatment of depression most often follows traditional psychopharmacological and psychotherapeutic paths. Electroconvulsive therapy
was the therapy-of-choice prior to the discovery and development of the
antidepressant drugs, but its use has declined as the convenience, ease,

and variety of drugs increased markedly. While these psychoactive drugs have made spectacular progress in allaying the symptomatology of depression, and have found widespread usage, it remains clear that adequate comparative research appraisal of differential effectiveness of the enormous wave of new drugs is lagging far behind their use (Beck, 1967).

Psychotherapeutic methods of relieving depression have been tried over a longer period of time than drugs and differ from chemical treatment by stressing the importance of determining the psychodynamic basis for the patient's problems rather than providing relief of the presenting symptoms. In most kinds of psychotherapy a mixture of supportive and insight methodologies is employed. Therapists seek to assure the depressed patient that the symptoms of his afflictions will disappear in time (as they do with most patients), they probe the life situation of the patient to permit him to ventilate his feelings, they suggest beneficial changes in the life situation or environment of the patient, and they attempt to modify the pressures with which the patient is failing to cope.

Cognitive or insight therapies may also rely on reassurance and catharsis in dealing with depressed patients, but these are preliminary steps en route to the final goal of reorganization of the patient's thought processes and insight about the reasons why he reacts with depression to conflicts others resolve more comfortably. The depressed person is considered the victim of proneness to react sensitively to the affronts of life with idiosyncratic cognitive patterns fashioned originally in childhood and thus poorly adapted to adult circumstances.

Probing into past events in the life of the patient, "insight" therapists search for those developmental experiences that may have sensitized the patient to respond selectively to certain types of experiences (Beck, 1967). This careful review of personal history has as its aim uncovering the stresses that produced a maladaptive response to life's conflicts. Hopefully, insight about these formative features in psychic life will allow the patient to evaluate current and future situations in rational rather than emotional terms. The depressed person, such theorists insist, must learn of cause-and-effect in his personal life if he is to short-circuit maladaptive responses in the future.

Electroconvulsive methods of treatment can also lift depressions even though the reasons for improvement remain a mystery. Psychopharmacological methods, too, remove the symptoms of the moment but offer little promise of improved response to pressures or mature reactions to conflict-laden life situations while the patient is free of drugs. For all its time-consuming, expensive, and complicated features, psychotherapy yet offers the most thorough-going means of dealing with current depression and warding off onsets of self-attack in the future.

Recently, behavioral therapy has been used to treat a number of neurotic disorders. But, this method has singularly neglected depression as a target for attack. In part one can explain this, as Lazarus (1968) does, by the vague and imprecise criteria used to define depression. Until this disorder is clearly delineated, he reasons, the behavioral-learning methods of treatment can have little impact. Time will tell, of course, but it is possible that the best of desensitization and conditioning techniques may have little impact on the ego problems depression represents.

SUMMARY

The depressive reaction is a mood change marked by severe feelings of helplessness and hopelessness and retardation in physical activity. Following a social or personal failure or interpersonal loss, the depressed person regresses and is unable to cope with anxiety about his worth and lovability as a person. If the depressive reaction is sufficiently thorough going, the patient may think of taking his own life to escape from the intolerable anxiety. For some, attempted suicide is a dramatic appeal for help; for others it is an action of last resort when personal psychological resources have been exhausted. There are a number of possible dynamic explanations of suicide, and a common thread of self-punishment runs through them. The depressed person feels guilty about having failed to be the kind of person significant others in his life can love. Traditional psychotherapeutic attempts to give the depressed patient insight into the source of his negative feelings about himself continue as a standard technique. But, the proliferation of psychopharmacological drugs in recent years means that most depressed persons in our society will be treated with some chemical mixture of psychic energizers, stimulants, or tranquilizers.

Hysteria and Psychophysiologic Reactions

HYSTERIA

The ancients were without an adequate theoretical explanation for hysterical phenomena, yet they made sense of it as best they could by reference to devils and evil spirits. In the late 19th century the neurologist Charcot began a systematic study of hysteria, but he could not free himself of the then current physiological theorizing and chose to believe hysteria was a hereditary degenerative process that directly influenced the central nervous system. When Charcot found himself face to face with clear psychogenic evidence about the origin of this disturbance, he yet maintained that it reflected some invisible, underlying physiological condition. In essence, Charcot failed to cast off the bonds of the theoretical system to which he was trained.

With Bernheim and Pierre Janet the next plausible steps were taken. Bernheim was a medical practitioner using hypnosis as a convenient ancillary technique; he saw hypnosis and hypnotizability as normal characteristics of human beings rather than as indications of an underlying disease process. His contemporary—the more theoretically oriented Janet—accepted a full psychogenic explanation, yet even he would have felt more comfortable with a physiological explanation of the witnessed events. It required a Sigmund Freud to elaborate the theory of hysteria and the steps in this process are worth reviewing.

Freud and Hysteria

In the early 1890's a relatively young, brilliant neurologist, Freud, spent some months working in Charcot's clinic. Impressed by the absence of a reliable neurological basis for most hysterical symptoms, Freud returned to Vienna and abandoned neurology to begin a fruitful collaboration with Dr. Josef Breuer and to study the intricacies of neurosis. In 1895, Breuer and Freud published the first important psychoanalytic document—*Studies in Hysteria*. They discovered that hysterical symptoms would disappear if, during hypnosis, the patient could recall the precise circumstances in which symptoms first occurred and could ventilate those emotions originally experienced. The release of these suppressed emotions and the expression of these pent-up feelings, which Breuer labeled *abreaction*, led to a "cure."

However, Freud began to encounter some difficulties with hypnosis. He did not particularly care for the method and was not a good hypnotist. In addition, some patients resisted hypnosis and others failed to benefit from curative suggestions. As an alternative, Freud asked his patients simply to relate to him (without censorship) whatever thoughts came to mind. He then discovered that patients could not easily obey the fundamental rule of telling all their thoughts and associated ideas even when they were convinced that this method could resolve the distress they were suffering. The patients seemed to resist the cure. Freud reasoned that the forces at work producing *resistance* must be part and parcel of the very forces which had banished the painful thoughts and feelings from consciousness in the first place. To protect the personality from a disturbing encounter with anxiety, shame, guilt, and lowered self-esteem, repression removed certain emotionally charged experiences from consciousness and was effective, despite therapy, in maintaining the status quo.

Freud began to think that the trouble with his hysterically neurotic patients lay in the hidden memories or reminiscences which were finding expression in symptomatic form. Freud proceeded to ask himself what thoughts, feelings, or experiences could be so fearsome as to require repression. Considering the mores of the citizens of Vienna in the late 19th century, he concluded only sex could provoke so much anxiety. This conclusion was neither unexpected nor novel, since the general medical practitioners of that era had long suspected there was a meaningful relationship between nervous disorders and the sexual life of patients. The term hysteria, for example, was coined by the ancient Greek physician, Hippocrates, who attributed the disorder to an absence of sexual stimulation that caused the womb (hysterus) to wander to various parts of the body. Marriage was the "cure" Hippocrates suggested.

When Freud codified and elaborated these ideas into a scientific position, he scandalized his colleagues by making a number of observations about adult and infantile anxiety. Freud observed that: (1) The sexual need is active in infancy and, to a lesser degree, throughout childhood. (2) Sexuality in childhood is more diffuse than in the adult and may take the form of (a) thumbsucking, (b) exhibiting the naked body, (c) curiosity about the bodies of others, (d) masturbation, and (e) pleasure connected with anal excretion, retention, or any stimulation of the erogenous zones of the body. (3) Sexual impulses are not innately attached to any particular object; object choice is learned. In childhood, therefore, members of the family, playmates, or adults of either sex may become the object of sexual expression. (4) Childhood sexuality provokes active adult disapproval which tends to encourage repression of the impulse. (5) Childhood sexual experiences, fantasies, and repressions exert a powerful effect on overt sexual behavior at puberty when the methods of satisfaction and object choices must be established if a normal sexual life is to be accomplished.

In the initial phase of Freud's theorizing, neurosis was the outcome of conflicts over sexual needs which were at first opposed by society (or its representatives in the form of parents, church, state, laws, and institutions) and later opposed by the part of the self that became identified with, and incorporated, the values, prohibitions, and regulations of the parents and society—the super ego.

Freud dealt with what he thought were two other distinct groups of patients—neuraesthenics and anxiety neurotics. The patients in the first group had symptoms of fatigue, listlessness, constipation, headache, and gastric upset. Those in the second group were victims of periodic attacks of anxiety, nervous uneasiness, and dread. Freud thought both conditions were due to abnormalities in sexual life. He attributed the symptoms of neuraesthenia to excessive masturbation or nocturnal emissions and he felt anxiety neurosis was due to sexual excitement or stimulation without adequate outlet or discharge. He based these erroneous conclusions on a welter of anecdotal material gathered in interviews and, since he was convinced that both disorders had a somatic component, he concluded, as we noted earlier, that anxiety neurosis and neuraesthenia should be labeled *actual* neuroses while hysteria and the obsessions would more properly be called *psycho*neuroses. One should, he argued, diagnose neuraesthenia only when the symptoms were accompanied by a history of excessive masturbation.

Freud's major clinical interest was in the psychoneuroses. The so-called actual neuroses soon ceased to be active objects of study for Freud and, as a consequence, they are rarely mentioned as a significant part of modern psychiatry. Research and extended clinical experience have modified Freud's first conceptions of the origin and nature of hysteria and neurosis. Modern views of the dynamics of hysteria draw heavily on the careful observations of Freud, but they have advanced beyond his original views.

The Dynamics of Hysteria

When free floating anxiety is converted into physical symptomatology, we have the psychological reaction that was once called conversion hysteria. On the basis of the extensive evidence provided by battle casualties in World War II, the diagnostic label "conversion hysteria" was modified to read "conversion reaction" and the dramatic physical involvement characteristic of this psychic state was used to differentiate it from other neurotic patterns. The hysterical patient reacts with less than usual concern about his crippling symptoms—he seems rather to accept them with a kind of fatalistic ease and grace—and seems free of the anxiety the average human being would feel about such severe physical problems.

At this juncture it should be mentioned that the classic forms of hysteria rarely occur today. It is difficult to know whether this has come about because diagnostic practices have altered over time, symptom patterns have shifted in an accommodation to changes in our societal structure, and "fashions" in symptoms have come to hold sway, or whether these kinds of sensory distortion have actually declined.

Theorists have suggested that the psychoneurotic person whose symptoms reflect a conversion of unconscious anxiety into somatic complaints is reacting to environmental stress by gratifying his basic need to be dependent on others (as all sick persons are) and to withdraw from the competitive demands of the real world. This syndrome is reinforced by social mechanisms in our culture that provide compensation for such persons, e.g., pensions, damages for injury, and a newly defined social role can reward the hysteric undergoing a conversion reaction and make the semi-invalid state profitable. Our society has, in fact, produced many of the stresses that force immature persons to choose this level of response over more mature attempts to cope with adversity.

Shapiro's (1965) observations about the hysterical style of life suggest that more than simple repression is needed to account for the full dynamic range of hysterical behavior. Shapiro concludes, for example, that the hysterical personality is fashioned in childhood when a particular form of cognition and memory is learned. If cognition and memory are acquired in ways that make repression (or forgetting) an easily available means of dealing with conflict, a basic framework may be established for an adult life that views the world in impressionistic and diffuse terms. Lacking a normal fact-oriented, sharply defined perception of the real world, one would make repression the defense of choice that would be used in an excessive fashion in response to the strains and pressures of daily life.

The individual growing to maturity with this kind of cognitive equipment may apply little precision or focus to the facts and realities of living, be highly subject to the influence of others (i.e., be suggestible, impressionable, responsive to every fad and fashion of the moment, or easily distracted by each new stimulus that comes along). When thought processes accumulate impressions rather than factual material, they tend to provide powerful emotional reactions to life at the cost of logic and a rational appraisal of persons and circumstances.

An additional characteristic of the hysterical neurotic style is the unrealistic, incurably romantic, idealized, emotion-laden relationship to people and the environment. Oblivious to reality, the hysteric reacts in a sudden, emotional, global manner that is free of the normal complications and contradictions that most of us must consider when making judgments. In Shapiro's (1965) words, "[hysterics] are struck by things: and what these people see are the immediately striking, vivid, and colorful things in life. By the same token, the simple factual details, the less obvious aspects, the contradictions, and the dry, neutral weights and measurements of things tend to be absent from hysterical notice. The subjective world that emerges in this process is a colorful, exciting one, but it is often lacking in a sense of substance and fact" (p. 119).

From this life view may emerge the "histrionics" of the hysteric, i.e., the theatrical, play-acting sense of unreality so characteristic of his behavior. This exaggeratedly unconvincing emotionality is not a pretense; it is a style of life in which the hysteric is unaware that he (or most often, she) is overreacting to stimuli. This fantasy-like way of life may lead to hysterical emotional outbursts that are offensive to others but barely noticed by the hysteric. Since such outbursts seem a reasonable and natural response to excessive provocation, their occurrence seems a part of the proper order of life. The indifference to their plight reported by those with conversion hysteria seems matched to the indifference with which they greet their own excessive emotionality.

The essential observation of Shapiro refers to the development of a cognitive and emotional style that provides the psychic setting for hysterical response to the problems of living. Shapiro's theoretical observations do not contradict analytic assumptions with regard to repression of unacceptable feelings and thoughts; they, rather, complement them by describing how hysteria can become a style of life.

Hysterics convert anxiety into physical disorders that may, symbolically, represent those impulses the individual must bar from consciousness, i.e., the body tells of conflict denied by the conscious mind. Once physical symptoms are formed, the psychic apparatus need no longer fear the unexpected appearance of unwelcome anxiety. Hysteria uses the body to express, symbolically, the impulse and the conflict it produces—eyes fail to see what they don't wish to view, ears can't hear disturbing information, and bodily paralysis prevents the individual from acting on impulses he cannot accept as a part of himself.

The body is a convenient vehicle for emotional expression. Hysteria is one source of bodily involvement, but it is not the sole basis of physiological difficulty. Psychosomatic disorders may also directly reflect psychological pressures.

PSYCHOPHYSIOLOGIC REACTIONS

The American Medical Association and American Psychiatric Association have listed psychophysiologic disorders as a separate entity falling, in their system of nosology, between psychoneurotic and psychotic reactions. Gregory (1968) refers to these disorders as psychophysiologic, autonomic, and visceral problems produced by an exaggerated state of normal physiological expression of emotions coupled with repression of the subjective feelings that usually accompany them. This definition suggests that the focus of this emotional disorder is on the transmission of psychological stress from the brain to the viscera by means of the autonomic system.

The simplest statement of the relationship of physiological reactions to emotional stimulation has been made by Levitt (1967): "The physiological responses to emotional stimulation are *autonomic*. The function of an autonomous response is to make an automatic, internal adjustment in the body without a conscious or voluntary effort by the individual. There are two kinds of autonomic responses: the *sympathetic*, the function of which is to activate body processes, and the *parasympathetic*, which acts to conserve bodily resources" (pp. 91–92).

Powerful emotions normally act on the body to increase the heart rate, elevate the blood pressure, speed up the pulse, improve the rate of flow of blood to the musculature, and stimulate the breathing rate.

At the same moment, the blood flow to the intestines, digestive system, and skin is decreased.

The antagonistic actions of the sympathetic and parasympathetic nervous system usually maintain the human organism in a relative state of equilibrium, but sudden, strong emotions force an imbalance that favors readiness for action and response. This steady energizing of parts of the nervous system and associated organs is both ennervating and physically destructive if it is continued over a long period of time. When we speak of psychosomatic events, then, we are referring to how the individual manages anxiety and we are suggesting that a learned predisposition to be anxiously aroused in a variety of situations is typical of persons victimized by psychosomatic complications in their lives (Lazarus, 1966; Spielberger, 1966).

The Dynamics of Psychosomatic Disorder

Consideration of psychophysiologic disorders requires some discussion of what has been called the mind-body problem. While this issue may, today, seem to be of purely academic interest, its consideration will give us a necessary perspective for understanding the logic and reasoning of the theorists who first put forward notions of psychosomatic illness. The nature of mind-body relationships has long concerned thinkers who have probed for the essential nature of man and sought to unlock its mysteries, and this is an important chapter in the development of thought about the neuroses. In part consideration of this issue is important because the untold reaches of new discovery in the natural sciences may well alter some of the traditional conceptions we hold dear about the nature of emotional disturbance.

There are roughly three theoretical approaches to the issue of the relationship of mind and body (Kaplan, 1967; Nagler, 1967). Double aspect theories insist the mind-body problem is primarily a semantic issue caused by the use of such terms as mental or bodily to describe the same phenomena simply viewed in different ways. Another theory, psychophysical parallelism, holds that mental and bodily processes are independent but run a course parallel to one another. For the average person, there is a preference for an interactionist theoretical view in which the mind and body influence one another but are distinct aspects of a single process, existence.

The interaction of mind and body is a complicated affair involving a complex hierarchy of physiological control mechanisms most of which are only partly understood (Treisman, 1968). There is seldom malfunction in a single system; any alteration of physiological function necessarily has a spread of effect throughout the other parts of the interlocking networks that make up the human body (Sternbach, 1966). Until we one day disentangle these elements, we must rely heavily on speculation and assumption to explain psychophysiologic symptoms. Often, the best we can do is to indicate the main systems or sites of the body that seem involved in particular psychophysiologic disturbances (e.g., cortical, endocrinological, midbrain, etc.).

As Kolb (1968) says, "Cumulative problems of interpersonal relationships produce a large share of the tensions and anxieties that beset the human being and upset physiology. Lack of emotional satisfaction in one's life may act likewise. Anxiety reactions to situational difficulties and crises seem particularly prone to be expressed in psychosomatic symptoms" (p. 414). Sickness can be, thus, a reflection of the attempt to solve unyielding problems of human relationships.

When anxiety becomes a bodily rather than subjective emotional experience, we say the individual is somatizing. Exactly how this occurs is a matter of continued conjecture. Is there specificity, i.e., are psychosomatic disorders a specific form of bodily response to particular conflict or are they nonspecific bodily responses to anxiety and stress? Is a target organ selected by the interaction of hereditary inclination and environmental stress, or is the choice of symptom location an unpredictable accident? For modern theorists, it is evident that some combination of predisposition on the part of the individual and precipitating stress in the environment is needed to produce this incapacitating bodily response to anxiety.

It was hoped that clinical research would one day uncover a specific personality profile to match exclusively each psychosomatic condition (Dunbar, 1946). Research in the two decades that followed made it clear that the body can be used as a vehicle for expression of personality distress in a great variety of psychiatric diagnoses (Holland and Ward, 1966). Failing to discover any simple relationship of conflict and disorder, researchers turned to an examination of multiple factors that might upset the homeostatic physiological balance and produce disorder (Lidz, 1959). This direction led inevitably to a broad concern with the full range of patient personality and problems of living.

Rough personality profiles can be used as a means of organizing facts about persons with psychosomatic disorders if we include in such descriptions an account of the psychological stress that provokes the reaction, the conflict and anxiety that occur when stress is dealt with inadequately, and the reaction of the person to awareness of his physiological distress (Alexander, 1950).

Unlike the symptoms of conversion hysteria, the psychosomatic or psychophysiologic reactions involve actual changes in the anatomical structure or physiological functions of the body. An hysteric activates response in organ systems that are manipulable by voluntary, conscious control; the psychophysiologic reaction involves organ systems that are under the control of the autonomic section of the nervous system and cannot, normally, be triggered voluntarily. Another important difference is that hysterical physical symptoms do not jeopardize human life in the way that psychophysiologic disorders can.

When the body responds in a destructive manner to one's inability to manage the emotional, social, and psychological aspects of life, the primary focus of psychosomatic disorder is in the internal organs and can be traced to malfunction of the digestive system, skin, muscles, blood pressure, heart, and breathing rate. The outcome of these malfunctions is apparent in peptic ulcers, neurodermatitis, ulcerative colitis, muscular pain, anorexia nervosa (compulsive vomiting), asthma, and migraine headaches.

It is important to note that theories about the dynamics of specific cases may be accurate appraisals of a particular individual's psychic condition yet not applicable universally to all persons manifesting roughly the same kinds of symptoms. There is an unfortunate tendency to assume that the dynamic conditions of a very few apply as well to all asthmatics, ulcer victims, or hypertensives. Disorders of determinable psychogenic origin are uniquely individual dynamic happenings that are never duplicated precisely in another person even when the symptoms appear identical. And, there are at least two kinds of allergic disorders (physical sensitivity to some allergenic substance and allergic reaction at times of psychological stress) and it is not easily possible to detect the source of the disorder by observing the symptoms alone.

The judgment that symptoms predominantly reflect psychological stress can only be made following an often lengthy and detailed scrutiny of the natural history of the individual.

Psychosomatic disorders may severely limit one's adaptation to life yet be the only resolution of oppressive forces the person can manage. The individual does not make a conscious decision to be sick, he simply does the best he can (given the circumstances) and psychosomatic complications are the outcome. As Cameron (1963) notes, psychosomatic disorders are adaptive since they may protect the individual from an even worse fate, i.e., the alternative to psychosomatic distress may be a psychic breakdown of a serious sort—as serious, perhaps, as psychosis.

The Varieties of Psychosomatic Disorder

The victim of a psychosomatic disorder is a sick person who acquires all the benefits of care and concern by others that usually accrue to such a role. The role of sick person varies, of course, with the organ system "chosen" as the vehicle for expression of the anxiety that is kept from conscious awareness. We can examine a representative sample of psychophysiologic disorders in order to add concrete details to our understanding of this means of managing anxiety.

Cardiac Reactions

Most of us are anxious about the condition and functioning of the heart since its failure or malfunction is so final. Under stress, the heart rate and blood pressure increase and rhythm of the heart beat may be altered to produce an "effort syndrome" in which fatigue, heart palpitation, headache, shortness of breath, and tremor of the extremities may appear. Awareness of these symptoms can stimulate additional anxiety which can, in turn, produce complicating additional symptoms of apprehension, restlessness, sweating, and depression (Whitehouse, 1967). The individual reacts "as if" he is engaged in heavy physical effort, even though he is sitting quietly, and this effort syndrome can easily be traced to anxiety about possible cardiac malfunction.

Concern with cardiovascular disorders must include consideration of the malfunctions of circulation of the blood through the body called essential hypertension. The physiological mechanisms that produce cardiovascular complications are nearly identical to those involved in hypertensive reactions. These partly understood physiological mechanisms defy precise formulation, but they are known to be triggered by stress and conflict. In the hypertensive, these physical conditions do not reach the damaging level attained by those with cardiovascular damage but the feature of constant threat is always evident (Alexander, 1950; Dunbar, 1946; Weiss and English, 1957).

Any of a number of emotionally charged situations may trigger vascular reactions that result in hypertension and complicate the reaction to the symptoms when they appear. Although there exists a variety of physical bases for elevation of blood pressure, in the bulk of cases of hypertension no clear physical reason can be discovered (Kalis, Harris, Sokolow, and Carpenter, 1957). Nor are we certain of the exact contribution of heredity (Miall and Oldham, 1963) or environmental circumstances (Pickering, 1965) to this order. Thus, a clear picture of the genesis of hypertension is still exceptionally elusive. Most hypertensives will receive symptomatic treatment rather than psychotherapy and never learn why they are responding in a physiologically excessive manner.

Continued hypertension can produce clinical pathology in the heart, brain, and kidneys. Yet, the disease is usually benign, and a great many cases have been reported in which patients with unusually high blood pressure levels have led long, productive lives and died of diseases not directly related to hypertension. There is not always a direct relationship between the symptoms of hypertension (breathlessness, headache, dizziness, fatigue, etc.) and high blood pressure readings (Reiser, 1967). Most of these symptoms have been attributed to psychological sources (e.g., concern about one's blood pressure). Clinical observations of hypertensive patients suggest there is an undercurrent of common personality and a similar pattern of adjustment among them. Hypertensive persons are often reported to be dependent on others, anxious to please, and quite unassertive despite the presence of unexpressed, critical, and hostile feelings toward others. If the hypertensive person could be inveighed to permit himself an emotional outburst and express the long suppressed resentment he has felt, the theoretical assumption would be that his blood pressure would decrease, and he would feel better (subjectively) if he could manage the guilt such an outburst would occasion.

This kind of clinical theorizing about hypertension is typical of a number of psychological "explanations" of physiological disorders of all kinds. Such conclusions about the personality make-up of patients are so frequently based on unscientific, limited, and impressionistic observations that the validity of these dynamic formulations is quite questionable.

As Reiser and Bakst (1959) have observed, cardiovascular difficulties become psychological problems ". . . not only because of the role of emotional forces in contributing to clinical disorders of the circulation but also because circulatory disorders, in themselves, frequently constitute sources of psychologic stress for patients and create problems in this sphere. Particularly in patients with heart disease (and to almost as great an extent in patients with hypertension), these psychological problems in reaction to the physical disorder are frequently more intense, and hence more serious, than the generally encountered reactions to the 'threat of illness' in a non-specific sense" (p. 659).

The stress occasioned by real structural heart disease can, thus, trigger somatopsychic problems in which the patient's care and treatment is complicated by a high level of anxiety about congestive heart difficulties. Some patients react in a maladaptive fashion to the fact of heart disease, convalesce exceptionally slowly following corrective surgery (Kennedy and Bakst, 1966), or invalid themselves despite medical advice that urges them to moderate activity. Often too, the mere diagnosis of possible heart problems can trigger a host of symptoms that were nonexistent prior to the diagnosis; the diagnosis of probable difficulty stimulates visions of sudden, inelegant death that are disproportionate to the actual threat.

And, real physical limitations are reacted to as if they were much more severe than they really are.

The recent success of heart transplant surgery has complicated the situation in interesting ways. Some of the first transplant patients are reported to have reacted negatively to their new physiological lease on life by denying the operation has actually taken place, suffering incapacitating anxiety about the prospect of physiological rejection of the new heart, or prolonged convalescence. Pioneers are always exposed to anxieties most of us will never experience, and we can feel sympathetic to the plight of the heart transplant recipients and acknowledge the reasonableness of this kind of reaction. Still, excessive concern with heart function does not occur for all such persons and we must again note that the personal patterns of reaction must be dealt with in psychological terms.

Research has yet to specify the exact characteristics of a "coronary personality" (Mordhoff and Parsons, 1967) or to provide us with reliable signs of impending coronary disease before it strikes (Poffenburger, Wolf, Notkin, and Thorne, 1966). By the same token, we cannot outline clearly the personality characteristics of persons with essential hypertension.

Headache

Psychophysiologic disorders involving musculoskeletal reactions that take the form of headache are an exceptionally common means of managing emotional distress (Friedman, 1967). A headache is a legitimate excuse for nonparticipation in tension-producing or distasteful aspects of life since it incapacitates the individual so effectively. In addition, there are secondary social gains that are induced by a splitting headache. Not only is an anxiety-provoking social or professional situation avoided, those close to the victim lavish solicitude and care on the headache sufferer.

A severe headache can also be a tool used to manipulate others—a means of managing one's relations with others. The case of Marge S. is illustrative of this situation.

MARGE S.

Having a headache that would force Marge to retire from the world of people had its origin when she learned she could get away with it. Marge's mother had always been overly concerned with Marge's health and would make a great fuss, not only when Marge was actually sick, but even when Marge looked like she might be coming down with something. Marge regularly had Monday morning sicknesses that kept her home from school. These maladies had a high correlation with academic stresses such as examinations, or scheduled performances of any sort in school. Marge had learned to alert her mother to possible illness early in the game. She would complain of a vague pain or of the beginning of a patterned set of symptoms but would dismiss these as inconsequential as soon as her mother became concerned and began to cross-examine her about her physical condition. This move on Marge's part established several premises: that she was about to come down with something, that she was prepared to suffer it through heroically and without complaint, and that only a severe attack of some dread disease would keep her from meeting her responsibility. Her mother played the game according to these unspoken rules, and Marge soon learned that there was profit in sickness if it was used wisely and adroitly. With practice, Marge became expert (McNeil, 1967; pp. 76–77).

The most common kinds of headache are caused by muscle contractions and by vascular spasm that usually encompasses the forehead as well as the back of the head, neck and shoulders. This pain is usually the result of continuous, strained contraction of the muscles in this area (Wolf & Wolff, 1953). At least 15 different kinds of headache are known to exist.

Respiratory Reactions

As long ago as the ancient Greeks there was speculation about the relation of emotional states to asthmatic attacks. In a classic instance, a patient allergic to roses (judged by her asthma attacks in their presence) suffered an identical attack when confronted with a papier-mâché rose. Similar cases have been recorded in which the predictability, regularity, and periodicity of the attacks makes emotions rather than allergens the suspected agent. What begins as an allergenic response may soon have a learning or conditioning process impressed on it in such a way that the psychological cue is enough to trigger the physiological response (Turnbull, 1962).

For many individuals, however, sensitivities develop to a number of allergens in nature and the reactivity of the person becomes a continuing source of difficulty (Freeman, Feingold, Schlesinger, and Gorman, 1964; Herbert, Glick, and Black, 1967; Jacobs, 1966; Rees, 1959).

Respiration is the single bodily activity that comes under both voluntary and involuntary control of the nervous system, and it is a process for which the infant, instinctively, does not need help from others. If oxygen is not inspired and carbon dioxide not expired, death results, and this frightening fact makes respiratory difficulties beautifully subject to psychological complications. As Witthower and White (1959) suggest, "Laughing, crying, sighing, pain, anger, fear, and sexual excitement have respiratory and emotional components which are inseparable. Talking, with its variations in pitch, inflection, and volume, may be an important respiratory expression of feeling states. Finally, contemplation of physical activity, particularly in the presence of real or imagined danger, is known to be associated with increased respiratory activity in anticipation of increased metabolic needs" (p. 690). In the primitive spectacle of the child holding his breath in an attempt to wrest from the environment the pleasures it seems to be withholding from him we see one version of use of the body to express rage, frustration, irritation, and discomfort. Adults don't indulge themselves in so obvious an expression of emotion, but they can subtly alter the function of their respiratory system while unaware that their body is speaking the silent message of their mind.

In bronchial asthma there is a physical constriction of the bronchioles of the lung and choking, gasping, and wheezing is commonplace. Not all bronchial asthma is caused by psychogenic factors, of course. Some asthmatics respond to real physical allergens in the environment. Certainly some conditioning of the individual to allergenic-laden environments must occur whatever the source of the incapacitating illness. At best we must conclude that a complicated series of factors contribute to the production of asthmatic symptoms. The body is a machine caught up constantly in movement and internal activity, and when one aspect of its functioning is disturbed, alterations in adjustment may occur throughout those systems closely and distantly connected to it.

With asthma, local cellular damage to the bronchioles in the lungs is thought to render its victim ever more susceptible to attacks in response to some environmental allergen. This would be a simple diagnostic and therapeutic problem were it not for the fact that symptoms vary in an unpredictable way. There are, thus, at least two kinds of allergic disorders: those responsive to some antigen-antibody interaction and those responsive to psychological stress. Theories about respiratory complications based on emotional difficulties have reached far afield to include susceptibility to the common cold, excessive smoking, bronchitis, pneumonia, and post-nasal drip. But, there is no logical reason to interpret *all* physical disorders in psychogenic terms even if the speculations are accurate for a few disturbed individuals.

In bronchial asthma emotional forces may play a predominant part. With or without some inherited responsiveness or inclination to asthmatic reaction, individual emotional conflicts are known to contribute to the disorder. The fundamental psychodynamic considerations for Witthower and White (1959) include an inordinate need for maternal dependence and love, an ambivalent attitude toward the mother, and fear of losing or destroying the mother. Exploration of these psychodynamic postulations have, unfortunately, been based on too few cases, too much theoretical speculation, and too little reliable, experimental evidence.

A usual clinical explanation of recurrent asthma traces it back to childhood and the nature of the parent-child relationship (Fitzelle, 1959; Margolis, 1961). Clinicians who deal regularly with asthmatic cases describe the "asthmatogenic mother" as of the following types:

1. The "deprived" mother who is anxious, self-pitying and has only meager personal resources to offer to the child.
2. The "achievement" oriented mother who has high personal aspirations for herself and equally high goals set for the child.
3. The "assertive" mother who is impulsive, controlling, and oriented to the use of power.

In clinical-experimental work exploring these types of mothers of asthmatics (Block, Harvey, Jennings, and Simpson, 1966) reasonable evidence was uncovered only for the "deprived" mother. The excessive responsivity of asthmatic children (Hahn & Clark, 1967) to a variety of stimuli in the environment has required particular care in therapy (Knight, 1968) and has uncovered the fact that removal from the home or separation from the home environment produces dramatic improvement in some, and steady improvement in most, children (Ford, 1968).

Therapy

Ideally, we would hope both the psychic and somatic aspect of psychosomatic difficulty would be considered in treatment. The fact is that this condition is most often unrecognized by the general practitioner, and when the psychic component is recognized for what it is, it too is usually managed by a liberal application of tranquilizers or sedatives. In those instances in which the emotional basis of physical disorder is clearly evident, a combination of physical and psychological therapies should be applied. In severe cases—cases that prove to be intractable to the usual physiological medicaments—psychotherapy should be used.

Often, however, the urgency of the physical symptoms is such that medicine takes priority over probing for the psychological basis of the disorder. The difficulties of maintaining the psychotherapeutic relationship are many in number and, most often, the patient's prime anxiety is focused on his physical symptomatology and he only begrudgingly deals with its psychic component. The physical symptoms are so central a concern to the patient that his motivation is less than adequate to the demands that will be made on him in therapy. Too, improvement in his physical condition is often the signal for a "flight into health" and the abandonment of the psychotherapeutic relationship.

In addition, psychotherapy is impeded by the many secondary gains that are accorded an illness that is sufficiently handicapping to reduce the competitive pressures of life. The immediate social gain of being sick augers poorly for a heavy motivational investment in psychotherapy. Therapy, then, must be adapted to the presenting circumstances in each individual case and medication may need to be used before rapport is established between the patient and therapist. In time, however, the family setting and environmental pressures must be explored if permanent relief from symptoms is to be accomplished (English, 1967; Meissner, 1966).

SUMMARY

Hysteria, in which bodily symptoms appear without an adequate neurological basis, was attributed by the ancients to the wandering of the womb throughout the body in the search for sexual gratification. This early observational connection of sexuality and hysterical reaction was confirmed in Freud's theorizing and has remained a mainstay in psychogenic conceptions of the disorder. When anxiety is not attached to some object in the environment, it is labeled "free floating" but when it fails to reach consciousness and is converted into symptoms of physical disorder it is attributed to conversion hysteria. In the latter instance, incapacitating physical symptoms can be symbolic representations of conflicts that were never resolved during childhood development.

The hysteric represses awareness of those impulses and conflicts that would be socially censured or repulsive to the individual if they were to find open expression. When this defensive repression fails (the repressed returns), an additional defensive maneuver is called for and the forbidden impulse or unresolved conflict is "converted" into a physical disorder that frees its victim from conscious anxiety. With life-long practice, the hysteric may develop a style of life that can include a fixed and inefficient way of perceiving and understanding the events in which he or she is immersed, an incurably idealized romanticism about life, and addiction to playing a role in life rather than living with its reality.

Psychophysiologic disorders are produced when anxiety is not met head-on and coped with in a problem-solving fashion. These feelings of anxiety do not find expression in overt behavior. They are, rather, channeled into autonomic and visceral reactions in which the body reacts to pressures in personal and social life. Man's normal physical equilibrium is overturned and organ systems in the body are upset while one's conscious life remains tranquil, e.g., rage and resentment are not expressed to others but the stomach churns in an acid bath that produces, finally, a peptic ulcer.

While we have yet to uncover the exact details of the mind-body interaction, it is apparent that cardiac reactions, essential hypertension, headache, and respiratory reactions all may have an important psychological component that can complicate the onset, course, and recovery from physical symptoms produced on a psychosomatic basis. The secrets of psychophysiologic disorders may be the last aspects of psychopathology to be understood. And therapy for these complicated disorders will, for some time, remain exclusively medical in form.

The Neuroses and Therapy
6

Our prime concern has been more with the nature and characteristics of the neuroses than with the means of relief from them even though some observations have been made about therapeutic remedy when it has been relevant to a particular disorder. While it is beyond the scope and intention of this volume to deal exhaustively with the principles of psychotherapy, some additional comment about recent therapeutic developments may be helpful.

THERAPY TODAY

Psychotherapy

There are a number of ways of defining the purpose and goals of psychotherapy: (1) relief from anxiety, symptoms, and conflict; (2) establishment of personal maturity, a feeling of adequacy, and integration of the disparate parts of the self; (3) the improvement of interpersonal relationships; and (4) providing adequate adjustment to the culture and the society (Watkins, 1965). These psychotherapeutic goals are not mutually exclusive, of course, and the variety of means to these ends has grown steadily, e.g., supportive, reconstructive, hypnotherapeutic, recreational, reeducational, psychoanalytic, cultural, Gestalt, holistic, active, objective, analytical, client-centered, relationship, individual, experiential, psychobiological, existential, projective, release, narcoanalytic, and motivational. It is obvious that each of these therapies emphasized one approach to the exclusion of others. It is our confusion about how best to alter man's personality and character that has contributed to this proliferation of means to a common end.

Much of the present day approach to psychotherapy is derived from the theoretical principles espoused by Sigmund Freud. Classic psychoanalytic treatment methods focused on bringing unconscious motives and conflicts into conscious awareness in order to deal with them in an adaptive fashion. Insight about the unconscious basis of neurotic behavior was then translated by the therapist and patient into altered patterns of interpersonal relationships and personal behavior. Hopefully, the posttherapy life of the patient would then be characterized by a substantial diminution in regressive, distorted, and inappropriate responses to living.

Psychoanalytic therapy was devised to deal with neurotic difficulties, but its application since its inception has been restricted to a very few affluent members of the middle and upper classes. Typically, the neurotic patient in our society will be exposed to treatment procedures that can best be described as dynamic psychotherapy based loosely on psychoanalytic methods. Depending on the symptoms the patient is experiencing, it is likely today that some form of adjunctive chemotherapy will also be employed.

The psychotherapeutic relationship is usually a unique experience in the patient's life. The neurotic person discusses his most intimate and secret feelings, thoughts, and reactions with a professional helper who is accepting of the patient as a person—a person who analyzes behavior rather than criticizing or condemning it. The therapist looks at the patient's life through a set of trained and disciplined eyes, tries to help him understand the nature of his problems, and assists the patient in seeking to discover a new or modified style of life that will be more rewarding and personally comfortable. Essentially, the neurotic person is required to work through a productive relationship with his therapist. In the course of this effort, the inappropriate and self-defeating patterns of perception, cognition, feeling, and behavior are laid bare and the process of reconstruction can take place. Penetration of the defensive structure that has for a lifetime protected the patient against accurate self-analysis is then a first, vital task in therapy.

It is obvious that our burgeoning population has long ago outstripped the capacity of the limited number of trained therapists to deliver therapeutic help on a one-to-one basis. At best psychotherapy is a remedial effort; its aim is to repair the ravages of a lifetime of exposure to psychologically crippling experiences and conditions. Hopefully, our society will one day do more than pay lip service to the idea that we must change a number of social conditions known to contribute significantly to the formation of neurotic ways of responding to life and emphasize prevention rather than remedy.

It is utopian to think that clinical research will soon discover prescriptions for marriage, child-rearing, education, and interpersonal relations that will guarantee a conflict-free, undistorted course of life for all human beings. It is equally optimistic to hope our institutions will train enough psychotherapists to serve the growing needs of our population. It is clear that new approaches to the disorders of living must be developed—approaches such as group sensitivity training to be discussed in a later section of this chapter. In the meantime, the typical neurotic seeking assistance with his problems will most likely receive treatment from his family physician and this will take the form of chemotherapy involving some combination of tranquilizers, energizers, stimulants, or depressants.

Psychopharmacology

The psychoactive chemicals have found widespread use in our drug-oriented culture since they have proved to be a convenient and effective means of freeing patients from the imprisonment of their symptoms. Few practitioners would deny that the aim of the psychoactive chemicals is primary symptomatic relief rather than problem solving. The practical defense for this readiness to drug neurotic persons has always been that the patient, once free of his incapacitating symptoms, is in a better position to work through and alter the internal and external pressures in his life that contribute to his personal discomfort.

Yet, if our conception of the development of a neurotic style of life has any merit at all, it would seem reasonable to conclude that there is little likelihood that victims of neurosis would be any more capable of lifting themselves by their psychological boot straps when heavily sedated or tranquilized than they would be when experiencing a full range of distressing symptoms. It is logical to assume that just the opposite would be more likely to occur, i.e., the tranquil patient would have even less motivation to undergo the rigors of personal therapeutic encounter. Since drug therapy will probably remain the treatment of choice for neurosis for some years to come, it is worth taking time to describe the major features of most used psychopharmocological agents.

The most convenient, simplest, and probably least accurate way to conceptualize the new drugs is to sort the various chemical compounds in terms of their intended effect, e.g., tranquilizers and energizers. Since drugs alter the balance of body chemistry and it is this new physical equilibrium that brings about change in behavior, we can never predict exactly whether tranquilizers will really have a beneficial effect on a particular individual. Thus, treatment still requires a great deal of trial and error not only with a variety of drugs (each of which differs slightly from the next) but with proper dosage levels of a single drug or various drugs used in combination. The most common tranquilizers, for example, have both sedative and tranquilizing effects and it is not easy to distinguish one effect from the other (Holliday, 1965).

The tranquilizers in most frequent use today are derivatives of a chemical grouping of phenothiazines bearing trade names such as Mellaril, Sparine, Compazine, and Thorazine. These are described as major tranquilizers; the minor tranquilizers such as Miltown, Equanil, and Librium have very modest tranquilizing effects and are often used as a placebo (a sugar coated pill with no real therapeutic value beyond psychological reassurance) for patients whose anxiety is relieved by "doing something," i.e., taking medicine. These chemicals can be used to calm anxious patients (anxiety neurosis, essential hypertension, secondary anxiety about psychophysical disorders, etc.) or to produce a state of indifference to the existence of emotional problems. In some obsessive patients, for example, both the obsessive thoughts and compulsive actions continue, but the thoughts are less vivid and the actions less vigorously pursued. In some cases the symptoms remain in nearly full force but the victim ceases to be as concerned about their presence as he once was.

The sedatives (barbiturates such as amytal, nembutal, phenobarbital) are also used to diminish awareness of the psychological discomforts of daily life and to reduce the restlessness and agitation that accompany personal problems. Sedatives can be used to help the anxious individual manage some unusual emotional stress or interpersonal crisis since they are faster acting than tranquilizers. Sedatives can take effect quickly to produce the desired effect; tranquilizers must be ingested for some weeks before tranquility is achieved on a stable basis.

The energizers (or antidepressants) are designed to shift the mood state of the patient out of depression and back to a less hopeless frame of mind. This is accomplished by stimulating an increase in the general level of behavior (increased appetite, less awareness of fatigue, increased speed of action and reaction both physically and intellectually, less sleep needed, etc.). By triggering the brain to a new state of alertness, these chemicals help the depressed person to reinvolve himself in work and recreational activities and this involvement itself rekindles his interest in the outside world and makes the future look less hopeless. Antidepressant drugs have proved to be particularly useful for those persons who are not only depressed but anxious about this condition and anxious about the state of the world. The psychostimulants in most common use are Benzedrine, Dexedrine, and Ritalin.

It is difficult to evaluate the status of therapeutic intervention in neurosis in modern America for a number of reasons. First, traditional psychotherapeutic efforts reach only a restricted segment of our total population and a limited number of those in need of psychological help. Second, the average neurotic individual does not come to the attention of civil authorities as a consequence of bizarre or socially incompetent behavior. Third, neurotic reactions are most often treated by general medical practitioners who may be ill-equipped to make a proper diagnosis. Finally, the widespread distribution of energizing, tranquilizing, and sedating drugs may have produced a massive masking of neurotic symptoms, precluding any attempt to search for the causes of disorders. The problem is that the effect of neurotic behavior on loved ones and on each new generation of children may continue to be exerted whether the patient is tranquil or not. One day, we must return to dealing with the causes of neurosis rather than its symptoms.

THE GROUP SENSITIVITY EXPERIENCE

One of the most recent therapeutic innovations is the formation of voluntary groups of persons who gather together seeking insight into their personal lives by means of group encounter. A great many variants in technique have been used experimentally including nude therapy (the participants shed their clothes in order to reduce the normal defensive facade that is a barrier to communication) and marathon therapy (the group members stay in continuous encounter with one another over an extended, unbroken period of time). The form these group methods have taken and will take in the future need not concern us here. What is important is that people have formed groups spontaneously to seek their own means of assisting one another in the quest for greater maturity and freedom from anxiety.

For purposes of illustration we can discuss the approach being taken by T-groups and sensitivity training on college campuses across the country. The young people of the new generation see the group experience as one means of achieving greater insight, interpersonal honesty and openings in living.

During the college years, "normal" students, as well as those with a neurosis or personality disorder, are likely to come into contact with other students interested in forming "encounter" groups devoted to increasing personal insight and expanding sensitivity to others. Involvement in a "group experience" is an integral part of the psychological tenor of our times, particularly among those members of the younger generations who are struggling to discover authenticity in life and to define a meaningful social and personal self. Thus, there is an easy availability of these experiences on college campuses across the nation.

There is, too, an emotional, cult-like quality to such group happenings. The neurotic seeking an answer to the mysteries of a life he is managing badly may look to the group encounter for an easy solution to some very complex personal problems. For this reason, and because this trend to group encounter will probably escalate in the next few years, T-groups deserve a careful evaluation.

T-Groups—Their Goals

The modified educational technique or group therapeutic form of interaction called the T-group (T for training) is devoted to "sensitivity training" with essentially "normal" people—those who are not institutionalized and those who would consider themselves normal. The T-group experience is participated in, for example, by an untold number of business managers and executives each year in the National Training Laboratories in Bethel, Maine (National Training Laboratories, 1967). The methods of group sensitivity training have struck a resonant chord among some educators, psychologists, social workers, and humanistic philosophers who have used the technique in an attempt to redefine and rediscover the meaning of existence.

The goals of T-group training include increased self-insight and self-awareness, sensitivity to the behavior of others, expanded understanding of the factors that inhibit or facilitate group functioning, improved diagnostic skill in interpersonal and intergroup situations, new freedom in taking positive action, and greater depth in analyzing one's own interpersonal behavior. T-groups differ in the degree to which each stresses particular features of these general goals and in the methods or groundrules established for conduct of the group encounter.

T-groups typically employ face-to-face, unstructured encounters to achieve their aims—unstructured in that the trainer or leader actively avoids organizing the group, outlining its purpose, or defining means to group goals. Group structure and organization are expected to evolve from the interaction of the participants as they spontaneously discover how they view themselves (individually and as a group) at this moment in time, i.e., what is happening to this group, in this setting, as it struggles to define its course, purpose, and meaning. The ambivalent purposes and emotions of the members of a leaderless group become grist for the experiential mill. The anxious attempts of individual group members to organize and lead in unconventional or conventional directions then become events other members can analyze and react to. How this process finally achieves the goals set for it is discussed by Klaw (1961) and Kuriloff and Atkins (1966).

The theoretical underpinnings of the T-group method (Campbell and Dunnette, 1968) include the expectation that individual human beings will provide valuable and constructive feedback to one another when they feel psychologically safe in so doing. Theorists also assume that individuals can accurately assess, and agree about the interpretation of, one another's behavior. Other premises are that behavior in the group realistically reflects behavior that is likely to occur in the world outside; that strangers can learn to feel safe about revealing their secret, inner feelings to one another; that all of us can benefit from an expanded insight into ourselves and others; and that what is learned in the close confines of the group has practical applicability to the real world each participant has briefly left behind.

T-Groups—Their Effects

Whether the above assumptions are warranted and whether the expected outcomes of the T-group experience match the hopes theorists ascribe to them are questions that can be answered only by systematic examination of the elements of the process and the reports of personal effectiveness. Subjectively—if we can accept testimonial evidence as scientific—the overwhelming majority of T-group participants report that the experience has made a meaningful and significant contribution to their personal and professional lives. Only the most fanatic theorists would conclude that this experience could be unremittingly constructive and remedial to every participant; if it one day proves to be modestly effective with a substantial number of "normal" persons, sensitivity will be justified.

Research into the effectiveness of T-group experience is, unfortunately, less than adequate. This is not hard to understand since each T-group may differ from others in methods and goals and since no coherent, overriding position has achieved enough acceptance to bind together all the diverse elements of the group process. Clear, reliable tests of the degree to which T-group learnings are transferred to "back-home" settings pose an additional knotty research problem. It is fair to suggest that we remain uncertain of the exact extent of the impact on the day-to-day life of participants in such sensitivity sessions; it is possible that the game-like quality of such an encounter and the artificial conditions under which it is experienced may militate against transfer of learning to the hard reality of one's personal social and psychological situation. The research challenge is a complicated one and one that has yet to be grappled with in a vigorous fashion. Which personal attitudes, beliefs, and behaviors are significantly altered by the T-group experience? How do you measure the reality of such changes, and how do you disentangle T-group impact from the all-pervasive effect of a multitude of other pressures and forces in the participant's life?

Despite the acknowledged difficulty of obtaining reliable scientific assessment of the impact of T-groups on the personal and social life of its participants, a number of attempts have been made to measure the outcome of this method. As Argyris (1964) has noted, research on T-groups has not been especially plentiful in recent years. It is as if the underlying philosophy is oriented to experience rather than scientific measurement. After a comprehensive review of the research extant, Campbell and Dunnette (1968) have concluded that evidence of the ability of T-groups to induce behavioral changes "back home" is convincing but quite limited. Exactly what changes do take place is less than clear because of an unfortunate confusion of terms and technical labels. We are not yet in a position to specify the exact nature of the changes that ought, reliably, to occur following exposure to a group experience of unspecifiable dimensions. Thus, the bulk of research is limited to amassing individual testimonial appraisals of subjective estimates of the consequences of barely describable T-group experience. When reports of altered self-perceptions of the participants are explored in fine detail, the results are even more confusing and less reliable. We will not be able to predict alterations in "back home" response until we are able to state exactly how, and to what degree, each individual is changed by T-group training.

It would be helpful, for example, if T-group theorists could be more exact about specifying those changes participants might reasonably expect to issue from the experience, i.e., the kinds of group experience in which change might be expected to occur or the kinds of persons most susceptible to change. No sensible theorists suggest that any method will affect all persons equally or be as effective in one "home situation" as another. We need to know which part of the process has which effect on which life situation. T-group outcomes need to be compared with other forms of influencing human beings, and the exact nature of the experience of the individual and of his interaction with the group needs to be made explicit and measurable before we can draw trustworthy conclusions. We need to answer questions about the structure of T-groups, the time period, the setting, and the participants. In an era in which a variety of conflicting and competing methods are being tried, we must be cautious about dismissing innovations in an off-hand manner simply because they deviate from tradition; at the same moment we must curb our eagerness to treat the new as better without a mature evaluation of its worth.

T-Groups—Cautions and Questions

T-group involvement has had unique repercussions among graduate students preparing for participation in somewhat more traditional therapeutic approaches to bring about changes in human existence. At the University of Michigan, for example, some students preparing for a career in Clinical Psychology became heavily involved in "sensitivity training." In an amicable confrontation with this abandonment of traditional forms of clinical experience, the issue was explored jointly by faculty and students and the confrontation of new and old raised these issues about the state of the art:

> Even within conventional clinical practice, strategies that create a therapeutic climate for one patient may bolster the neurotic defenses of the next. However, we do have some rule-of-thumb criteria as to what constitutes intensive therapy aimed at individual character change. For example, a characteristic of most therapies, regardless of theoretical orientation, is the quality of *uniqueness.* In actual psychotherapy, the patient presumably encounters a therapist who is not part of his consequential social system, whose communications and actions are not predictable from the mores and conventions of the extra-therapeutic world. The patient is introduced to new modes of communication and conception, and hopefully to a new self. But, while the intent of T-group workers is to establish this same quality of uniqueness for the individual group member, it is in reality difficult to separate the styles of communication and leadership that are practiced in encounter groups from trends that are prevalent in the student culture as a whole. That is, encounter groups seem to extend, formalize, and at times deepen a style of discourse that is now very pervasive, across settings, for the kinds of people who are attracted to T-groups. Though there is no doubt inter-group variation in these terms, encounter groups strike the naive observer as a continuation of the vague philosophizing, the public introspection, and the obsessiveness in regard to affective matters that is the current student ambiance. Thus, T-groups do not seem to provide participants with new settings, with new styles of discourse and cognition, or with new *data.* The participants often know each other from other settings, introspection and the data of the internal life are no news to them,

and their goals often have more to do with expressivity than with insight. In the T-group, expression of affect seems to be an end in itself, and not a way-station to the usual clinical goal of symptom relief or basic character reformation.

In the therapies that we consider effective and try to teach, treatment and cure are judged in terms of ego capacities that the patient has developed for himself, with the help of the therapist, and not in terms of the *therapist's* development as "person," as a "whole man," or whatever, during the patient's tenure. But in encounter group work, it would be very hard to make this sort of distinction between client and change agent. In this culture, groups and individuals imply each other, such that individual growth is defined in terms of group development and *vice versa*. Thus, while T-groupers use some of the insights, models and especially the rhetoric of clinical psychology, they do not seem to use these as tools for fostering individual change, conceived as such, nor are they intended to foster eventual *autonomy* from groups and group process. The participant is trained to help create or to seek out the kinds of groups that will bring out his best capacities as a group member; he is not trained to live, if need be, *outside* of groups. Granting the possible virtues of this collective ethic in an age of alienation, it is hard to see how these enterprises could bring about autonomous inner development of the sort that is the usual goal of clinical practice. The collectivist perspective of the T-group world must be taken into account when we make judgments about the clinical import of one or another group practice. For example, in the group setting, self-disclosure and introspection do not have the usual "clinical" goal of bringing unconscious contents under ego control. For the group, these practices are more an end than a means; they are an enactment of the collective ethic. . . . The point is that most participants do not come to groups with the motivations and vulnerabilities that patients bring to psychotherapy. They are not usually in a state of anxiety brought about by the opposition of highly charged impulses and rigid defenses. Their problems have to do with alienation, rather than guilt; and they come to the group as a place where they will be taken seriously, on their own terms. Given these motivations, and these definitions of trouble and of remedy, it is not surprising that participants are not particularly troubled by group review of their character flaws and defenses. Their inner life is not particularly explosive; and they have some hand in creating the style and standards of the critique, even when it is used against themselves. At such time their problem has become the group's problem: they are being taken seriously; alienation has found its remedy. By far the worst trauma is to be ignored.*

This example of the conflict between T-groups and traditional therapeutic methods reflects the core issue of therapy and neurosis. While the limitations of classic methods are well known, and frequently criticized, the invention of new methods does not always assure us of a better means of undoing the ravages of developmental events that culminate long-standing alterations of personal adjustment.

What would be the most likely fate of exposure to group sensitivity experience for an anxiety neurotic, a victim of phobia, the obsessive-compulsive, the amnesiac, the depressive, or the person undergoing a psychophysiologic reaction? Without reliable evidence we can only speculate, of course, but it is the author's conviction that group sensitivity training was never intended, nor is it suited, to deal in depth with neurotic problems. If we are even approximately correct in our appraisal of the dynamic basis of neurotic conflict, it is evident that a group encounter could not penetrate a long-practiced defensive barrier or provide insight into the unique, personal circumstances of learning that have contributed to the distorted psychological makeup of the full grown person.

SUMMARY

Traditional psychotherapeutic approaches to neurotic disorders have had as their goal not only relieving the patient's symptoms but providing insight about the self-defeating reactions that characterize him in interpersonal relations. Most modern, dynamic psychotherapies are modifications of the form and theoretical principles of classic psychoanalysis. One-to-one therapeutic methods have, however, proved unequal to the needs of an expanding population that has grown sophisticated about the level of service it requires.

Most neurotic patients will not receive psychotherapy of the traditional sort; they will, rather, be seen by their family physician (who may fail to diagnose the problem properly) and will be given sedatives, tranquilizers, or psychic energizers (antidepressants) to remove the anxiety occasioned by the neurotic symptoms. In most instances, no adequate search will be made for the root causes of the person's neurotically disordered life.

A recent development in experimental approaches to psychotherapy

---

* Personal communication from Professor David Guttman, The University of Michigan.

THE PERSONALITY DISORDERS II

Personality

The growing child must master a series of accomplishments in the course of development. He must, as he grows, learn about people and must experience the real world; he should acquire the capacity to think, feel, and behave within a restricted range of socially approved dimensions of sensation, perception, thought, emotion, motivation, and verbal and motor behavior. Disorder in any of these aspects of social existence may prompt others to confine him, punish him, restrict his freedom, or discriminate against him. Implicit in this range of approved and disapproved social actions is the conviction that there are correct and incorrect, acceptable and unacceptable, good and bad ways to experience life (Forest, 1967).

This means man must learn to respond to his bodily sensations in ways that roughly match those of his fellow citizens. He must also think approximately in the way others do in order to communicate effectively with them. He must express emotion with the proper intensity and appropriateness, and his verbal and motor behavior must fit the public mold or he will be in social trouble.

The term personality has been used to describe a person's objectively observable behavior as well as his inner experience. These mixed public and private aspects of life have a number of adjectives attached to them to describe the individual, e.g., ambitious, religious, hostile, passive (Brody and Sata, 1967). These descriptive phrases are a kind of prediction of how a person will act in a variety of normal situations as well as a prophecy of the form emotional disturbance will take. Personality is formed developmentally out of the continuous interplay of the genetic and biological nature of a unique human being in interaction with people and things. It is in how one meets and responds to events and relationships that the shape of personality is cast. According to modern theory, most of this is accomplished in the early, growing years.

The perpetual compromise between internal drives and external demands produces patterns of behavior that may be ego-syntonic (experienced as a normal, natural part of the self) or ego-alien (experienced as strange and outside the self). Thus, some trait or personality disorders seem to the individual to be trouble-free, acceptable ways of living. In contrast; those suffering neurotic disorders may suffer symptoms that seem to be foreign, irritating, tension-laden, and anxiety-producing. The neurotic may be acutely aware of his discomfort and thus "self-diagnosing"; the person with a personality disorder may be so diagnosed only by others who are discomfitted by his way of life. Motivation for treatment among those with personality disorders or trait disturbances may be nonexistent.

Personality pattern or trait disturbed persons are those whose "life style demonstrates limited adaptive flexibility and certain relatively unchanging modes of expression and action . . . characterized by unsuccessful but repetitive attempts to establish a stable, reciprocal relationship with the environment; seemingly rational but actually self-defeating attempts to gratify needs; and restricted, sometimes inappropriate, and often stereotyped thoughts and feelings in response to highly diverse situations" (Brody and Sata, 1967; p. 939).

Once the limited collection of responses of such persons has been exhausted—and the problem or conflict remains unresolved—they may be forced to rely on crude, primitive, infantile patterns of reaction that are inappropriate to the problem of living they must solve.

Personality *pattern* disturbances are long-standing conditions that may, under severe stress, deteriorate into psychotic depression, paranoia, or schizophrenia. Personality *trait* disturbances are more circumscribed, limited aspects of the self that have their counterparts in normal behavior and adjustment. Personality trait disturbances are marked primarily by extensive immaturity and instability which may deteriorate under stress but are not likely to evolve into a full-blown psychosis.

The distinction between traits and patterns of traits needs to be made here. When we use adjectives to delineate human behavior (hostile, angry, etc.) we are describing a behavioral event that is likely to occur on a predictable basis. Several persons may possess the same trait, but the trait of each will vary so in strength, intensity, and regularity that they are discernibly different persons. A trait or series of traits can be assembled together to make a design or pattern that can then become characteristic of the individual. Not all traits fit harmoniously together, of course, and personality pattern disturbances may reflect exactly these conflicts.

Character and Type Theories

What we call *character* is a judgment we make about the features of enduring personality of ourselves and others—good character is what we approve and bad or disordered character what we disapprove (Allport, 1937; Michaels, 1959). An adequate theory of the nature of character formation and character structure does not yet exist since this aspect of human psychic existence has suffered both neglect and superficial treatment. In the early days of psychoanalysis there was an almost exclusive emphasis on neurotic symptoms, and Wilhelm Reich (1945) made one of the first attempts to fit the concept of character into the psychoanalytic framework. But this direction has been little pursued in modern times.

Reich and a number of other theorists roughly contemporary with him (Fromm, 1947; Horney, 1945; Kardiner, 1939) described character and personality types as a sort of capsule summary of patterns of human behavior. And this stimulated other theorists to try their hand at the ancient game of condensing the nature of man into brief, descriptive form. Havighurst and Taba (1949), for example, describe adaptive, submissive, unadjusted, defiant, and self-directive persons, while Riesman, Denny, and Glazer (1950), elaborating on some of Fromm's basic concepts, have delineated tradition-directed, inner-directed, and other-directed forms of social character.

Types and type theories have found little acceptance among clinical practitioners since these handy but inaccurate capsules are much too limited to contain the complexity of human beings. In addition, type theories evoke the image of rigid, unchangeable personalities. Most of us would resent being described in terms inadequate to encompass the complicated, variable, multi-faceted object we call our self. Whatever the current professional designation (character neurosis, character disorder, conduct disorder), there seems to be a consistent, identifiable core of behavior we call character. Clinicians deny the validity of type casting, yet they rely on it heavily in their daily work.

Personality Disorders in Childhood

In childhood, pattern and trait disturbances are clinically confusing since they occur in a human organism not fully formed. It is necessary to "stretch" the usual collection of diagnostic categories to fit children (Teicher, 1967). The more such categorization is forced, of course, the less meaningful it becomes. Current classification systems confuse us about the source, course, and treatment of childhood personality disorders. If a therapist believes treatment "X" should be applied to disorder "A" and disorder "A" is an inadequate description of the child's condition, only chaos can result. This statement is, of course, equally applicable to the emotional disorders of the adult.

If we had accurate developmental norms for each age, stage, and phase of human personality development we might be in a position to construct a coherent theory of the meaning of deviations from a norm. As it is, we can only continue to describe and classify as best we are able and hope our flawed attempt at systematization will one day evolve into a more accurate means of capturing the essence of personality. The American Psychiatric Association Diagnostic and Statistical Manual is not much help since it seems merely crudely to modify adult syndromes in a patchwork effort at fitting younger persons.

There is some hope in the labors of the Committee on Child Psychiatry of the Group for the Advancement of Psychiatry. Aware of the deficiencies of classification of personality disorders in childhood, this enterprizing group has suggested additional categories for personality disorder as follows:

1. ANXIOUS PERSONALITY—chronically tense and apprehensive.
2. COMPULSIVE PERSONALITY—excessive orderliness, conformity.
3. HYSTERICAL PERSONALITY—overly dramatic, flamboyant, emotional, seductive.
4. OVERLY DEPENDENT PERSONALITY—helpless, clinging, passive, dependent.
5. OPPOSITIONAL PERSONALITY—negativistic, stubborn, passive-aggressive.
6. OVERLY INHIBITED PERSONALITY—shy, constricted, passive, restrained.
7. OVERLY INDEPENDENT PERSONALITY—active, precocious, independent.
8. ISOLATED PERSONALITY—distant, detached, seclusive, withdrawn, emotionally cold, schizoid.
9. MISTRUSTFUL PERSONALITY—paranoid, distrustful, suspicious.
10. TENSION DISCHARGE DISORDER—aggressive or sexual acting-out, conflict with society, antisocial, sociopathic, or psychopathic conduct and/or behavioral disorder.

An additional set of refinements and subcategories might be included in this classificatory scheme, but the system continues to adhere closely to a descriptive categorization of childhood disorder with little speculation about the basic causes of the disturbances. This suggested system is a mixture of progressive (abandonment of adult syndromes as a model for children) and conservative (stay with description until more is known about personality development in children) points of view.

These diagnostic categories have not yet gained wide acceptance. At least it provides an additional perspective for the topics we are about to consider. The formal and official classification system of the American Psychiatric Association differs from that proposed by its Committee on Child Psychiatry as follows:

PERSONALITY DISORDERS [*]

Personality pattern disturbance
    Inadequate personality
    Schizoid personality
    Cyclothymic personality
    Paranoid personality
Personality trait disturbance
    Emotionally unstable personality
    Passive-aggressive personality
    Compulsive personality
    Personality trait disturbance, other
Sociopathic personality disturbance
    Antisocial reaction
    Dyssocial reaction
    Sexual deviation: specify supplementary term
    Addiction
        Alcoholism
        Drug addiction
Special symptom reaction
    Learning disturbance
    Speech disturbance
    Enuresis
    Somnambulism
    Other

The disorders of behavior produced by personality disturbance are rooted in significant events in childhood emotional development in which anxieties are produced—anxieties that can only be managed by defensive psychological maneuvers that take their toll of adequate adjustment. The disorders of character and personality have in common deviations in conduct that are censured, punished, and rejected by the controlling members of our society (White, 1964).

The neurotic patient experiences, typically, a series of internal frustra-

[*] American Psychiatric Association, 1952.

tions, conflicts, and symptoms. Those subject to personality and character disorders "act out" their difficulties by inflicting them on others in violating the code of social behavior by which most of us abide. The neurotic may have suppressed and repressed too much of his impulse life to adjust satisfactorily; the individual with a personality or character disorder may have suppressed or repressed too little to make him acceptable to his fellow man.

Let us look now to the forms that personality and trait disturbances may take. In the following chapters we will consider sociopathic disturbances, sexual deviations, and addiction to drugs and alcohol.

Sociopathic Personality Disturbance

8

The designation "psychopathic personality" was a favorite among therapists and theorists for a number of decades, but it was abandoned in 1952 by the American Psychiatric Association. As a category it was simply too all-inclusive to be useful (Hoppe, Molnar, Newell, and Land, 1967) encompassing as it did sexual deviates, gross inadequacies of character, schizoid and paranoid persons, and those displaying antisocial behavior (Cleckley, 1959). Psychopathic personality was submerged in the new nomenclature under the broad category of "personality disorders." Thus, the psychopath became a subdivision of "sociopathic personality disturbance, antisocial reaction" but he remains, as described more than a century ago, an asocial, aggressive, impulsive, guilt-free person who misbehaves socially and is thought to be without the capacity to form lasting bonds of affection to other people.

When clinical workers encounter a psychopath in a mental hospital, they are never quite certain he belongs there. As Halleck (1967) observed, "Even when we agree that he is a legitimate object of psychiatric scrutiny, we have difficulty in deciding what to call him. . . . The term 'psychopath' seems to be retained because it has communicative value" (p. 101). The psychopath is marvelously adapted to certain stressful circumstances and this makes it difficult to diagnose him with any degree of success. As Halleck says, psychopaths may function successfully in combat, in athletics, in amorous adventures, in challenging frontier settings, or, for that matter, in mental hospitals.

While the mythical pure psychopath may not exist in reality, there are some persons who closely approach a fit to this classification. Psycho-

93

paths seem able to function free of true emotional involvement with others and, having little regard for the needs or feelings of others, the psychopath may appear more cruel or aggressive than the average. But, this may be a consequence of his lack of concern about erecting the polite social facade that is socially common. The psychopath is not only unable to form close emotional bonds with other persons, he avoids much complicating entanglement.

Halleck has also observed that the psychopath's evident freedom from guilt may be a misjudgment the rest of us make when we observe a hedonist intent solely on seeking pleasure here and now without the regard we think he or she ought to devote to the past and the future. The daring, guilt-free, ahistorical psychopath intrigues those mortals among us who are less free of the well-learned lessons of socialization. Most of us envy, admire, and hate the few who seem to have the freedom we long for. The threat to society posed by the psychopath is that if a majority of us were capable of leading a life similarly free of care and anxiety, the organized elements of social life would suffer a devastating blow. We suffer, then, a powerful inclination to declare the psychopath or sociopath sick and to deal with him accordingly.

THE SOCIOPATH (PSYCHOPATH)

The newborn infant is a sociopathic personality since he can't tell right from wrong, is without feelings of guilt, and is controlled primarily by limitations in the outside world rather than by an internalized moral code. An infant uses others solely for his own gratification, and parents strive to change this state of affairs through selective reinforcement (reward and punishment). If the parents fail in this task, the child may well grow up to be a sociopath—an emotional infant in an adult body.

A number of lists have been constructed in the attempt to delineate the fundamental characteristics of the adult sociopath or psychopath. Coleman (1964) has assembled one of the most widely read summaries of symptoms (based on the observations of Cleckley, 1959; Darling, 1945; Heaton-Ward, 1963; Thorne, 1959; Wegrocki, 1961; Wirt, Briggs, and Golden, 1962). His list of characteristics includes:

1. Inadequate development of a conscience.
2. Low frustration tolerance, poor judgment, egocentricity, impulsivity, and irresponsibility.
3. The search for immediate gratification coupled with absence of long-range goals.
4. An absence of sufficient anxiety or guilt for self-control.

5. An inability to learn from previous impulsive actions.
6. Charm and a sense of humor used to exploit others.
7. Social relationships without love, depth, or loyalty.
8. Hostility toward, and rejection of, authority.
9. Lack of insight into his behavior.
10. A source of continuous difficulty for those close to him.

Buss (1966) describes the symptoms of the psychopath using a somewhat different list of characteristics. He emphasizes three vital facets of the psychopath. Psychopaths, as Buss describes them, are a kind of living-dead, i.e., they are isolated emotionally from other human beings and are without the ability to give or receive love as most of us know it. They may imitate and mimic human emotions, but it is a crude imitation of the tender feelings that produce loyalty or attachment to others. The psychopath has little in the way of a stable identity of his own since he cannot establish goals and values independent of the social advantage they will bring. Nor can he plan a life based on insight, responsibility, and a self-image derived from an objective view of himself in relationship to others. He gives nothing of himself to others; he takes from others to satisfy his needs.

Most important, he is impulsive, undisciplined, and cannot trade ephemeral and immediate gratification for more stable but distant gratifications. He does what pleases him now and lets the future care for itself. In this sense, the psychopath is stuck in the present and is incapable of dealing effectively with the future. He is one-dimensional; he does not learn from the past and he hasn't the patience to await the future. Immediate temptation is too compelling to resist even if it augers extreme loss in the future, and it is in this way that he is self-defeating. The case of Dan F. is a clear reflection of the attitude and world view of the full-blown psychopath.

DAN F.

Dan F. had married before, a fact he had failed to communicate to his present wife, and, as he described it, was still married only part time. He had established a reasonable basis for frequent nights out since his variety show required that he keep in touch with entertainers in town. He was currently involved sexually with girls ranging from the station manager's secretary (calculated) to the weather girl (incidental, based on a shared interest in Chinese food). The female of the "show biz" species seemed to dote on the high-handed treatment he accorded them. They regularly refused to believe he was "as bad as he pretended to be," and he was always surrounded by intense and glamorous women who needed to own him to feel complete as human beings. . . .

As we discussed his early life he told me he could not recall a time when he was not "doing everybody I could and the easy ones twice." He remembered that when he was 12 years old he had read a pocket book about "con men." It was then he decided it would be his life's work. They were heroes to him and he "fell down laughing" when they took some "mark" for his "bundle." As he said, "There is a sucker born every minute, and I'm glad the birth rate is so high."

When Dan was a teenager he was a model of recklessness and revolt against authority. He pressed for those illicit experiences denied the young and became what every parent feared was the shape his own child would assume. Even at that age he knew in his bones what behavior would comfort the anxieties of "old folks" and lead them to believe that their half-remembered impulses were not typical of the new generations they now had to comfort. He assumed that parents preferred a lie to the truth, so he was careful to be what they hoped him to be rather than reveal himself for what he really was. He became a skilled small-talk conversationalist as he submitted himself to the critical scrutiny that regularly took place in the dead time that existed before his date made her dramatic entrance into the living room. . . .

As he said, "I could con them the same as I fooled my own folks. When I got caught by the cops I always blamed the other guys. I would admit to just enough to make me appear to be a slightly imperfect but earnest kid who deserved another chance. They went for it time after time, not because they believed it but because they couldn't stand the idea that I was really a rotten kid. Mostly they didn't want to be bothered by it all. When I figured that out I didn't have to lie so much. They believed anything I told them because they didn't want to hear anything else and that way they got out of the messy deal quicker" (McNeil, 1967; pp. 85–86, 87, 88).

The sociopath, then, refuses to accept life as it is lived by others. He is blunted emotionally, indifferent to the feelings of others, and carries into adult life the characteristics we usually attribute to the spoiled child. His entanglement in the seamier side of life is predictable but often excused because of his intelligence, charm, and promise to reform. He is more interesting than most people but he is an expensive companion. He won't grow up and he can't be depended upon, but he is, on the surface, literate, bright, and charming. Perhaps he is what Cleckley (1955) accuses him of being: a psychotic wearing only the "mask of sanity."

Causation

We have a conflicting set of possible choices with respect to causation; we can look to biology, to psychodynamics, or to some combination of the two. In addition, a third element—the culture—could be instrumental in the production of psychopaths.

1. Biological

The explanation of the mystery of the psychopath most favored by theorists in the past was that of an inherited biological or constitutional factor. The search begun then continues today. Eysenck (1960), Silverman (1944), and Stott (1962) are among the searchers for evidence of some biological basis for the development of the sociopathic or psychopathic individual, but the experimental evidence from these and related studies is not sufficient to be convincing to most observers.

A recent biological or genetic explanation of crime is that of the chromosomal constitution of the criminal (Montagu, 1968). Most males have a chromosome structure labeled XY, but now and then chromosome abnormalities are found of the XYY, XXY, XXYY, or XY/XXY mosaic types. Thus, the chromosome structure XXY occurs in 1.3 of every 1,000 births. In the last five years a series of reports have noted that the percentage of chromosomal abnormality among prisoners convicted of violent crimes is unexpectedly high (Hunter, 1968; Nielson, 1968). Richard Speck, the murderer of eight nurses in Chicago in 1966, for example, is said to be an XYY.

Based on these observations, Montagu suggests that our society might take as a first priority chromosomal typing of all infants shortly after birth in order to detect XYY formations in time to undertake preventative measures at an early age. I think some words of caution might be valuable here. Chromosomal research of this variety is far from complete. Base rates of chromosomal abnormalities in the normal population are not yet well established, for example, and this makes it difficult to assess the importance of deviation. In addition, there are a number of characteristics other than violence associated with such abnormality —low I.Q., unusual tallness, etc. (Telfer, Baker, Clark, and Richardson, 1968).

Finally we must remember that almost all of the crimes of violence committed in our society are perpetrated by persons with perfectly normal chromosomal structures. And, no statement linking chromosomes to criminal behavior will make much sense if the environment and life experiences of the individual are not added into the cause-and-effect equation.

For some psychopaths there may be a mixture of biological and social causation, but a more likely hypothesis is that psychopaths *learn* to be the kind of adults they become. The notion of a constitutional psychopathic inferiority involving some hereditary weakness of the nervous system is without evidence to support it.

2. Psychogenic

At the base of many conceptions of sociopathic personality is the observation that such persons seem to lack appropriate feeling for other people. The question becomes, then, how disturbance in early human relations produces deviation in the adult's emotional life. Basically, the child must learn, in the absence of close affectionate ties or a proper basis for identification with the mother, to imitate the emotions others are expressing if he wishes to be accepted and to get what he wants. White (1964) sums it up nicely, "the neurotic craves human relations, the delinquent fights them, but the psychopath seems to be merely indifferent" (p. 372). Indifferent, yes—but adept at using these relations for his own purposes.

A classic description of the early psychological environment of the developing psychopath was written by Greenacre in 1945. She described a generalized set of circumstances that might include components such as a successful father who, although a community leader, is distant and frightening to the son and a mother who is little less than a "kept" woman—pleasure-loving, self-centered, indulgent. Parental affection in such a family might amount to "buying-off" the child via material indulgence. Concerned more with the child's external appearance than with what he masks within himself, his parents teach him to pretend, to protect the family reputation, and to appear to meet other's expectations. Charm becomes, then, an acceptable substitute for achievement and failure is easily excused, dismissed as unimportant, or blamed on others.

When developmental experiences set the stage for behavior that is not controlled by conscience or an internalized set of values, we have the makings of the sociopath (Bandura and Walters, 1959; Herskovitz, Levine, and Spivak, 1959; Weinberg, 1952). Evidently, emotional deprivation experienced at the time the child is most dependent on others for guidance may result in antisocial aggression even among members of the highest socioeconomic level in our society. When such deprivation is compounded by desertion by or absence of a parent early in the life of the child, the effect is most severe (Glueck and Glueck, 1950).

All sociopaths are not, however, of the same kind nor do they come from an identical environment. Frankenstein (1959), for example, sees the mother as the most powerful force in producing psychopathology. He describes the morally indolent psychopath, the brutally destructive psychopath, the egocentric psychopath, and the psychopath who borrows another's identity since he lacks one of his own. In each instance the mother—whether indulgent, punitive, rejecting, or absent—is a central force in shaping the growing child. Other theorists, Robert W. White (1964) for one, share this view of the importance of mother-child relationships in the formation of the psychopathic character. Over-indulgence, or under-indulgence, rejection by the parents, or the absence of a proper model for identification can contribute to the formation of hostility that manifests itself in sociopathic behavior as the child grows to adulthood.

O'Neal, Robins, King, and Schaefer (1962), for example, studied the parents of (1) sociopaths, (2) persons with other psychiatric disorders, and (3) normals. They found the fathers of sociopaths likely to be sociopaths too. It is obvious that such studies cannot disentangle heredity and environment and tell us if psychopathy of this kind is a learned or genetically transmitted disorder.

For some theorists, what happens in the parent-child interaction is less important than the consistency and predictability with which it occurs. When the world is a maze of random, unpredictable psychological events, the child may learn that it is only safe to grasp at whatever gratification the moment may afford. Behring and Bruning (1967) suggest that there may be a failure in the ability of the child to learn to form concepts without difficulty. If the developing child experiences cognitive failure of this sort, it may be that the psychopath's world makes a different kind of sense to him than it does to others.

A number of research efforts have explored the dimensions of psychopathy. Lykken (1957), for example, decided that the inability of the sociopath to profit from social learning might be attributed to an absence of the anxiety most of us learn in childhood. Comparing psychopaths with nonpsychopathic controls, Lykken concluded that psychopaths were less anxious than those not so diagnosed. The observations of Albert, Brigante, and Chase (1959), Karpman (1941), and Painting (1961) confirm these observations as do the experiments of Hetherington and Klinger (1964) and Hare (1965). Without anxiety we do not learn; with a limited anxiety we learn a little; with adequate anxiety we learn what is necessary to survive the emotional give-and-take of society.

Antisocial and Dyssocial Reactions

It has been fashionable, if not entirely accurate, to refer to the sociopath as a person totally free of anxiety (Cleckley, 1959; Lykken, 1957). Such has seldom been the case in theorizing about antisocial and dyssocial personalities—persons who seem to disregard social rules and regulations or to battle vigorously against them. For these individuals anxiety seems an important part of the motivation for their behavior.

A dyssocial reaction describes the behavior of persons free of marked personality disorganization who nevertheless disregard the laws of our society and lead lives connected with professional crime (Hartung, 1965). This group makes up only a fraction of the official delinquents who grow to adulthood carrying deviate codes of behavior learned in criminal homes and deteriorated neighborhoods. Murder, robbery, burglary, rape, and other forms of predatory warfare against law-abiding citizens are characteristic of the dyssocial person. Again, we are referring only to a small percentage of our population. Fortunately for our society, not all young delinquents become adult criminals (Stubble-field, 1967). While the delinquent subculture in our society is a prime source of supply for the adult criminal population, not all criminals are grown-up delinquents (Matza, 1965). The dyssocial reaction is assumed to be one without severe personality disorganization, but the ranks of criminals can contain the full range of neurotic and psychotic disorders as can any other segment of the population.

It has been suggested by some theorists that the form of the dyssocial reaction has changed over time and that our society has a rising frequency of crimes committed for thrills, as opposed to the profit motive of organized criminal gangs. Middle and upper socioeconomic class dyssocial reactions seem, for example, to be an increasing feature of the current social scene. The use of illegal drugs (LSD, marijuana), stealing without material need for what is stolen, vandalism, and defiance of the law are pursued by middle and upper class children as a kind of affluent expression of personal and social anomie. Defective child-parent relationships are not limited to the poor, and crime is not always correlated with desperate need or absence of material well-being.

The prefixes *dys* and *anti* attempt to describe the differences between these two subtypes of social reaction. One class (dys) is without the usual restraints on lawbreaking behavior; the anti's accept the restraints as real but fight against them. The dyssocial person fails to accept the limitations of social rules when those rules interfere with immediate gratification or the expression of an impulse; the antisocial person is in active rebellion against rules he cannot accept as reasonable or rational. The antisocial person is frequently a member of a subculture alienated from the larger culture and dealt with in a discriminatory and prejudicial manner. He, thus, justifies his disobedience by insisting he need not abide by the larger society's conventions (Freedman, 1967).

In contrast, the dyssocial person is in favor of the culture only to the degree that it meets his needs and gratifies him when he demands it do so. The case of Tim C. describes a subcultural, antisocial reaction that will illustrate how tenuous is this distinction between dyssocial and antisocial. Tim has learned well how to master that segment of society most immediate to him. His success has been costly, however, since it has been at the expense of full participation in the larger culture.

TIM C.

Tim C. was well built for a 15 year old. At five feet ten inches, and 165 pounds, it was convincing when Tim "leaned on somebody." Although he actually spent very little time fighting, he devoted most of his energy to talk of toughness, threats, and inducing fear in others. His conversation seldom strayed far from the topic of aggression, and I often had the impression that he was imitating a gangster movie. Partly, his size was his problem. If Tim had grown to be a scrawny, under-nourished young man, his dealings with others and his view of the world might have been quite different, and, perhaps, he would not have been victimized by situations from which there was no face-saving escape. . . .

Tim was particularly verbal one day and told me what it was like to live as his family did. With some feeling Tim reported,

You get kicked out of one place and you move a couple blocks to the next pig pen. One of my "uncles" gets a truck and we load up all we got and go somewhere else. After we dump the junk in the new joint, I cruise out cool on the street and look out for whose ass I know I can whip. I'm "bad," man. I'm mean. After I drag the street once, I know what's shakin'. I know who's big and who ain't and what's going on. I don't mess with the guys that can beat me till I find out who's chicken and then I try a couple of them. I move in slow but hard and the next day everybody knows. Then they know "mess with me and you die." Nobody pushes with me and nobody says nothin' about my mother. Man, you got to push or suck hind titty where I live. I don't suck no hind titty. That's all. They fool with me and they in a whole world of trouble. You a whitey. You don't know nothin' about it. You can go downtown any time and nobody says nothin' to you. I got the color and I can't go nowhere except with my own kind. You try it and see how you like it (McNeil, 1967; pp. 95, 101–2).

The complex of pressures and influences that theorists have suggested might produce dyssocial and antisocial behavior is best summed up by Martin and Fitzpatrick (1964). ". . . at one time or another, crime and delinquency have been explained on the basis of race, defective physique, climate, capitalism, feeble-mindedness, poverty, mental illness, lack of recreation" (p. 31). In one sense, behavior unacceptable to society needs no explanation if it is viewed as a particular means of integrating inter-personal relationships. Antisocial or dyssocial activity provides immediate gratification for needs and impulses while it allows the individual to express anger and contempt for a society in which he cannot find a place.

It is in "acting out" behavior—the translating of impulses into action without restraint—that the quality of sociopathy is most apparent (Abt and Weissman, 1965). Acting on impulse makes the individual unpredictable. And when the impulse being expressed is a violent or hostile one, the sociopath becomes a danger to society.

The acting out of the young is a predictable part of development (Josselyn, 1965). Adolescence is a time of change not only in sexual status but in a multitude of other needs, drives, goals, and desires. These changes must be managed by an adolescent ego that is not always adequate to the task. Adolescents not only act *on* impulse, they act *out* impulses and conflicts left unresolved from earlier periods in their growth and development.

Cameron (1963) tried to bring some order to the issue by differentiating three subgroups of sociopathic personalities. One class of sociopathy included those irresponsible and emotionally limited persons who keep getting into trouble yet suffer little anxiety about it. Another class contains the antisocial person who is in open and aggressive rebellion against society. Dyssocial persons best described as corrupt criminal types constitute the third class.

For Cameron, emotionally shallow, irresponsible persons are those without the ability to postpone gratification. And they lack the self-discipline needed to establish stable, responsible, interpersonal relationships or to follow the rules and customs of society when these rules require they postpone immediate gratification. Childish, immature, irresponsible, and superficial, their values are in conflict with those of the larger society. The psychopath may be a professional criminal obsessed by a deeply felt, emotional rebellion against the authority of society. Among dyssocial adolescents, usual dimensions of misbehavior include not only delinquency but drug usage, overt defiance of parental authority, and assaultiveness (Kulik, Stein, and Sarbin, 1968).

Admittedly, it is difficult to draw a clear distinction between the various types of sociopaths since they resemble one another in a variety of ways. Robins (1967) believes the "dyssocial reaction either does not refer to a psychiatric illness or has not been studied in a manner to differentiate it clearly from antisocial reaction" (p. 951). There is some question, for example, whether the criminal population of our country could really be described, exclusively, as dyssocial. Robins (1966) has made one of the most thorough follow-up studies of sociopathic personalities and has traced the relationship between childhood antisocial symptoms and adult antisocial reactions. His conclusions are clear. While not all antisocial children become adult sociopaths, not a single child in his study developed an antisocial reaction syndrome as an adult in the absence of antisocial symptoms in childhood. An early appearance of symptoms seems a necessary but not sufficient condition for the adult form of the disturbance.

That categorization of teenage delinquents is far from a simple matter is attested to by the British criminologist K. R. Wardrop (1967). He suggests that an adequate type system should include some reference to causation as follows:

ORGANIC—those delinquents suffering from brain damage.

GROSSLY DEPRIVED—those suffering early deprivation, parental abandonment, or institutional care during the early years.

EMOTIONALLY DISTURBED—those whose fully developed neurosis or psychosis is a prime factor in dyssocial actions.

FAMILY PROBLEM—those who are reacting to unsatisfactory relations with their parents.

SITUATIONAL—those whose delinquency can be attributed to the culture and a set of values which legitimizes delinquency.

VARIETIES OF PSYCHOPATHS

At this point it is evident that theories of sociopathic or psychopathic behavior tend to make conflicting claims and must stretch themselves considerably to encompass an exceptionally wide variety of behaviors. One recent attempt to reduce the number of theoretical contradictions offers hope that by further subdividing the concept of the psychopath we will be able to untangle the various theoretical threads.

Let us consider Arieti's (1967) explanation of the varieties of sociopath or psychopath. For Arieti, the issue is one of distinguishing between psychopathic traits that make up a basic human pathology and those psychopathic traits which are secondary manifestations of other psychological disorders. Arieti favors the following classification:

1. Pseudopsychopaths (symptomatic psychopaths)
2. True psychopaths (idiopathic psychopaths)
   a. Simple
   b. Complex
   c. Dyssocial
   d. Paranoiac

The pseudopsychopath has psychopathic qualities but they are an integral part of some other psychological disorder, i.e., character neuroses or psychoneuroses. The pseudopsychopath might better be described as a "hostile character." They appear to be psychopaths but are, in reality, neurotics.

In contrast, the idiopathic psychopath of the "simple" sort is a victim of powerful needs for immediate gratification whether or not this gratification is socially sanctioned. Plagued by ungratified tensions, the simple psychopath acts to achieve satisfaction with little regard for the norms of society. Impatient with the complicated series of acceptable social steps the culture demands, he may indeed react impulsively and without regard for the social consequences. Intellectually, he is aware of the risks he takes but gratification has, for him, become an emotional rather than a rational matter. The psychoneurotic crippled with apprehension about the future would resist such dangerous immediate temptations; the true psychopath would not. Unable to delay gratification, the person we call a psychopath would do the convenient thing: "It is easier and quicker to steal or forge checks than to work, to rape than to find a willing sex partner, to falsify a diploma than to complete long studies in school. Lying is a slightly more sophisticated way of obtaining satisfaction. The lie leads to immediate gratification, enabling him to enjoy, for instance, an undeserved reputation" (Arieti, 1967; p. 248).

The complex psychopath as described by Arieti is a sophisticated version of his simple counterpart. He asks not only how to get immediate gratification but he adds an intelligent footnote to the question, i.e., how to get away with it. In a choice between self-realization (power, money, pleasure, etc.) and social morality (delay, playing by the rules, concern with others), social morality always loses. The complex psychopath can delay putting needs into immediate action if such delay is absolutely necessary but he remains a ruthless, self-serving user of others for his personal gratification. In a sense he is a careful, calculating psychopath who uses whatever immoral means are called for to enhance himself.

A third group of psychopaths consists of dyssocial persons who were never properly socialized to the values, standards, and ethics of the larger society. Thus, the professional criminal or gang member would seem psychopathic with regard to behavior expected by law-abiding members of our culture at the same moment he would be considered normal by members of his special subgroup. The dyssocial person is not restricted to criminal gangs whose standards allow taking short cuts to gratification. History is replete with accounts of social and political groups whose behavior violated the usual standards of the society.

Arieti raises the obvious question of whether this group is a truly psychopathic one or simply a sociocultural phenomenon that occurs in every society. It seems reasonable to assume that both the psychological make-up of the individual *and* a particular sociocultural situation (the existence of a criminal subpopulation) are needed to produce the dyssocial psychopath, since only a small percentage of our populace takes this way of life.

The paranoiac psychopaths described by Arieti are a rarer breed since they are psychotic as well as psychopathic. As Arieti notes, "Whereas the dyssocial psychopath needs a group which will release his tendencies to act out, the paranoiac psychopath needs a system of delusions which allows him to act out and to justify his actions" (p. 261). He is a psychopath who has constructed a paranoid delusional system to justify his actions. Arieti describes Adolf Hitler as a classic example of this emotional disorder in that Hitler believed the Jews of the world were plotting to destroy him and were responsible for the problems of the German culture. This fixed paranoiac delusion allowed him to seek self-realization directly and immediately via war and wholesale murder.

Arieti's system of typing of psychopaths eliminates the awkwardness of trying to distinguish clearly between asocial and dyssocial types of behavior, allows us to include psychopathic behavior that is mixed with paranoid delusional symptoms, and seems to account for sophisticated and complex kinds of psychopaths who never seemed to fit the description of the simple psychopath. Our next problem is to decide what remedial therapeutic efforts might be effective in altering these patterns of psychopathic response.

THERAPY AND THE SOCIOPATH

Treatment of sociopaths is difficult and exasperating since they seem to have all the necessary equipment to join the society of adjusted human beings yet they consistently, and seemingly irrationally, fail to measure up to reasonable expectations (Greenacre, 1945). The patient himself is of little help since he views his condition as an acceptable or even a superior way of life and rarely seeks or accepts assistance from those intent on "helping" him. Because the sociopath does not experience severe anxiety or intense feelings for other persons, the traditional levers for therapeutic manipulation are absent, and progress along usual lines seems impossible. Treatment of psychopaths by classic psychotherapeutic means has seldom succeeded (Cameron, 1963). In despair, some psychotherapists have concluded that treatment of the true psychopath, homosexual, paranoid, or drug addict is hopeless (Gibbons, 1965).

Hendrick (1958) reports results of psychotherapy that are quite discouraging (in one study, 22 out of 23 were unimproved). Total therapeutic communities (Jones, 1953; Kiger, 1967) have been established in an attempt at rehabilitation with varied success. Recently, Bernard and Eisenman (1967) have made attempts to reteach basic values to sociopaths using conditioning techniques; additional attempts have been made to teach patients useful self-controls (Greenwald, 1967).

The essential therapeutic obstacle is as much methodological as it is the condition of the person. Most verbal psychotherapies are best suited to the problems presented by anxious neurotics painfully aware of their discomfort, avidly seeking help, ready and willing to talk, and convinced of the efficacy of this method in producing change. In contrast, the psychopath views the world with a distorted vision and responds to others impulsively and with an eye to his own advantage. It has been suggested that therapy might best resemble a kindergarten in which emotional reeducation takes place, since it is an absence of moral learning that is suspected. All such attempts at "retraining" the psychopath seem, on the surface, bound to fail since an adult is no longer a helpless, dependent infant or child.

The treatment of sociopaths by other means has followed a variety of paths. Darling and Sanddal (1952) reported some improvement following psychosurgery, and Green, Silverman, and Geil (1943) used electroshock with limited success. A drug normally reserved for epileptics (Dilantin) has also been used to neutralize antisocial behavior (Silverman, 1944) for limited periods of time.

There is no chemical that can instill a conscience or socially-appropriate set of ethical values in an adult. By the same token, we have been unable to devise the means of inserting, in later life, what should have been learned many years ago. Despite the regularly recurring suggestion that we devote all our efforts to early detection and prevention of these conditions, behavioral science has yet to develop the know-how or tools necessary to such detection. Perhaps the psychopath will always be with us in one form or another. He exists now, he often is entrusted with social power, and he certainly will be a part of the social scene in the predictable future.

SUMMARY

Some in our society become adults alienated from the rules and regulations of social living by which most of us abide. The most intriguing form of this disturbance is the seemingly normal person who has grown to adulthood without the restraints that direct the behavior of the majority of us (conscience, judgment, tolerance of frustration, long-range goals, anxiety and guilt, insight, and emotional depth).

It is superficially easy to understand the antisocial depredations of the deprived, disenchanted, alienated person raised in a socially decayed part of our society—he seems to have a reason for his actions. It is harder to comprehend the antisocial rebel and the sociopath who was without material deprivation in his early years. Yet, we continue to produce a small percentage of the emotionally "walking-dead" among us. Somehow, parent-child relationships produce an early malignancy that grows to full size in the adult. We are not certain if this is a purely biological or a mixed biological-psychogenic state of affairs.

Therapy with sociopaths has been uniformly unrewarding. All known treatments have succeeded with some, just as all known treatments have failed with most.

The Sexual Deviant

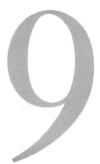

To be deviant one must depart from the accepted standard of behavior dictated by one's culture. But, deviant sexual behavior violates a complex social code that fluctuates exceptionally from person to person and group to group. Private sexual behavior, for example, so regularly conflicts with publicly approved actions that the meaning of deviation is obscure. The lay person's view of what constitutes sexual deviation does not match that of the clinical worker who must deal with human emotional disorders. It is only when sexual activity is "compulsive, exclusive, destructive, or accompanied by much anxiety and guilt" (Lief and Reed, 1967; p. 259) that clinicians get concerned.

Buss (1966) suggests three criteria for sexual abnormality: discomfort, inefficiency, and bizarreness. The typical sex deviant may be efficient in the conduct of his life and may feel no discomfort. Yet, the bizarreness of his behavior (as judged by others) might be sufficient grounds for labeling him deviant. We are each trained from childhood to follow socially approved patterns of sexual behavior and deviations from this standard are considered bizarre, i.e., the choice of an inappropriate sexual object, means of sexual gratification, or aim of sexual gratification.

Sexuality is such a fundamental part of the fabric of the total personality—inseparable from what we are to ourselves and how we are viewed by others—that to refer to sex is to speak of the whole person. Adult sexuality refers not only to the biological fact of sex but to sexual identity (one's sense of maleness or femaleness), gender identity (the social and psychological aspects of behavior related to being male or

108

female), and gender role (strong, active, dominant versus soft, passive, and submissive).

When a man assumes the role proper to his gender (he takes the male role) but with another male, it is called homosexuality. By the same token, the female who takes the female role with another female as an object is considered homosexual (lesbian). Sexual inversion occurs when the man reverses his role (is passive) with another man or when a woman assumes the masculine role with another woman.

At least among college men and college women, sex-role stereotypes continue to match despite social changes in the direction of greater permissiveness. We have taken legal steps to bring equality between women and men, yet both attribute greater social desirability to masculine characteristics. The social changes we have witnessed over the years have evidently not yet penetrated the consciousness and value system of the bulk of the young males and females in our college population (Rosenkrantz *et al.*, 1968). The appearance of equality seems to occur more rapidly than its emotional acceptance. It will probably require an alteration of child-rearing and socialization practices in the direction of less emphasis on the differences between the sexes before both social equality and equal value are placed on feminine characteristics.

We can define deviations in the physical world (differences in height, weight, length, etc.) in simple statistical terms, but norms of sexual behavior are not so easily or reliably measured with yardsticks of a length we can all agree about. Most often what is normal in sexual behavior is judged by local civic authorities in terms of personal conviction about what is proper (as their beliefs dictate) coupled with what is frequently an erroneous view of what the "average" person in the community believes. These subjective judgments about the moral standards of others have again and again been rejected as an adequate guide by the courts of our land.

Deviation and perversion are popularly defined in so many vague and varying ways that we cannot overestimate the value for our culture of the pioneering studies by Kinsey and his associates (1948, 1949, 1953) in opening the topic of sex to public discussion and in expanding the limited, local definitions of what is or is not permissible.

However, there are rough conventions of normal versus deviant in widespread use, and we can detail some of them here. A quarter of a century ago the material below would have been entitled "sexual perversions" (Stoller, 1968), would have borne a powerful moralistic tone, and would have categorized sexual preferences as right or wrong. The forms of sexual deviation most usual in our culture are not notably different from those that have existed since the beginning of time.

THE NATURE OF DEVIATION

The public makes a subjective judgment that a person who commits a bizarre sexual offense must be unable to restrain himself (as a "normal" person would) and must therefore be sick (Halleck, 1967). Such a person, although defined by society as sick, is rarely treated with the kindness usually accorded the sick. Our laws proscribing sex offenses are not only the most vague of all laws addressed to criminal behavior, they are the most irregularly and arbitrarily enforced. The forms of sexual deviation catalogued in Table 8-1 divide deviation into categories of intensity or frequency of sexual behavior, the mode by which sexual satisfaction is attained, and the objects chosen for sexual activity. These divisions, while arbitrary, will provide a perspective for our examination of the facts and theoretical approaches to sexual deviation that follow.

TABLE 8-1.   FORMS OF SEXUAL DEVIATION

Deviant Intensity and Frequency	Deviant Sexual Modes	Deviant Sexual Objects
Impotence	Oral-Genital	Homosexuality
Frigidity	Anal-Genital	Lesbianism
Nymphomania	Masturbation	Incest
Satyriasis	Sadism	Bestiality
Promiscuity	Masochism	Fetishism
	Exhibitionism	Pedophilia
	Voyeurism	
	Transvestism	

This means of dividing forms of sexual deviation is both awkward and somewhat misleading. Thus, for example, oral-genital contact is not considered a sexual deviation by most psychotherapists if it takes a heterosexual form and if it is a means to sexual stimulation rather than an end in itself. Masturbation, too, could easily be included in the section devoted to deviant sexual objects since the self is the exclusive target of the sexual response. It should be noted that most of the deviant modes of sexual expression are those that occur in heterosexual rather than homosexual contact. Thus, this list is a convenient if imperfect way to consider the topic of sexual deviation.

Theoretical Explanations of Sexual Deviation

For Halleck (1967) there are three broad theoretical explanations of the motivation for deviant sexuality:

1. Some sensitizing event during development that creates fears of heterosexuality.
2. The desire for forbidden and, thus, stimulating sexual activities, i.e., a desire for variety.
3. Deviation as a consequence of the influence of distorted parental relationships.

If we accept the notion that one *learns* to be homo- or heterosexual, then we would look to problems such as confused sexual identification, the search in later life for love denied by the father (in the case of male homosexuality), or the attempt to be masculine or feminine to fulfill unconscious parental needs. Psychoanalytic theorists believe sexual deviation results from the failure of the individual to make proper progress in mastering the developmental psychosexual stages that begin with the diffuse sexuality of infancy and end, ideally, with conflict-free adult genital heterosexual relationships (Apperson and McAdoo, 1968).

Deviant behavior (with the possible exception of a frequent association of patterns of voyeurism and exhibitionism) is usually specific to one form of outlet. The dynamics of each disturbance differ subtly depending on the nature of the emotional and behavioral experience of the individual. And it is suggested that the more bizarre the deviation, the more pathological the general adjustment of the individual. Brancale, Ellis, and Doorbar (1952), for example, report an unusually high proportion of personality disorder among those arrested for sexual offenses. In their study of 300 sex offenders, fewer than 15 percent would be described as normal, 10 percent were psychotic or borderline psychotic, and an additional 35 percent were severely neurotic. The degree of disorder was found to differ approximately with the form of deviation. Let us turn first to the deviations of intensity and frequency.

Sexual Deviation—Intensity and Frequency

Deviations in intensity and frequency of sexual response include impotence, frigidity, nymphomania, satyriasis, and promiscuity. The disturbances of impotence and frigidity make the members of our competitive, achievement-oriented Western culture exceptionally anxious. Impotence in the male, for example, may be a condition related to the characteristics of the sexual object which he prefers or with whom he happens to have intimate contact, related to the degree of sexual inhibition he is experiencing, or related to the fear and anxiety he feels about demands the female makes on him for potent performance. Symptomatically, the male may fail to achieve or maintain an adequate erection in sexual encounter or he may suffer ejaculatio praecox in which orgasm is experienced prior to, or just at the initiation of, sexual experience (Redlich and Freedman, 1966). Any or all of these events are, for males, disastrous for his sense of self-esteem.

Frigidity in females can range from difficulty of arousal and/or disinterest in sexual relations, to sexual intercourse without response, and to positive rejection of sexual advances of the male. Male anxieties that culminate in impotence may be matched by female revulsion at the prospect of the sex act. This revulsion in females may be based on fear of pregnancy, perception of males as animalistic "users" of the female, guilt about sexuality, or envy and jealousy of the social privileges accorded the male in our culture.

It is clear that emotional conflict, psychological distress, and severe anxiety find an elaborate, complicated, and convenient arena of expression in sexual encounter. When interpersonal relationships deteriorate or prove difficult, deviant sexual responses may be the first indication that problems exist. The disorders labeled nymphomania in females, satyriasis in males, or promiscuity in either, are one end of the continuum of sexual response reflecting emotional and psychological distortion. Thus, the need for continuous sexual encounter with a variety of partners on an obsessive and compulsive basis is considered a sexual disorder despite the fact that frequency and intensity of sexual experience is judged right or wrong on a very relativistic basis. When sexual encounter bears the unmistakable flavor of obsession or compulsion it, as any behavior, is judged pathological. When the intensity and frequency of sexual encounter are complicated by neurotic problems, the behavior ceases to fit anyone's description of normal.

Promiscuity should be considered a separate and special case. To define sexual behavior as promiscuous we must be able to determine the difference between a lot, a little, and too much. Such measures of degree obviously can only be relative to particular persons, in a particular society, at a particular moment in time.

When patterns of sexual behavior that differ from the usual form of coitus serve as the major or exclusive sources of sexual gratification (rather than an integral part of or as foreplay to, sexual intercourse), we label them sexual deviations (Friedman, 1959). Such deviations include the substitution of parts of the body (other than the genitals) as a primary source of sexual gratification or the focus on other than genital activity as a sexual outlet. Deviant sexual acts are considered "normal" if they are an essential part of heterosexuality; they are defined as psychopathological when they become an exclusive source of gratification.

Deviant Sexual Objects

When objects of sexual gratification are other than members of the opposite sex, we have the deviations of homosexuality, lesbianism, fetishism, incest, bestiality, and pedophilia.

Homosexuality

Historically, the frequency of homosexuality has varied from era to era within every culture in history. Those who defend homosexuality as a superior way of life regularly make reference to the sanctioned male-to-male relationships that existed in ancient Greece, but to put this era in perspective it must be recalled that early Greek society was historically one of the very few that endorsed homosexuality and that this cultural practice was based socially on a conception of the female as inferior to the male. The female was a species without the blessings of a soul (Churchill, 1967). Women were used for reproduction and male objects employed for pleasure, but homosexual contacts in those days were graded by age and status—the elder male making sexual demands on the younger male who was required to play the feminine role. Free expression was allowed for various forms of the sexual impulse in the culture of that time. And, for Freud, this latter fact—the emphasis on the impulse rather than the object—was all-important as an explanation of the mixed choice of males and females for sexual pleasure.

Based on the Kinsey, Pomeroy, and Martin (1948) studies of (self-reported) homosexuality, it is estimated that only 4 percent of our current population is exclusively homosexual despite the fact that between one-third and one-half of the males in our society have had at least one homosexual experience (usually a brief encounter in adolescence) in their developmental years. These homosexual experiences were most often an adolescent substitute for not yet obtainable heterosexual objects. About 10 percent of males are exclusively homosexual for about three years between the ages of 16 and 65.

Homosexuality that is repressed and never appears in clear-cut overt form is described as latent homosexuality and may only be apparent in secondary forms—interests, hobbies, slight mannerisms, etc. (Bieber, 1962, 1967). The concept of latent homosexuality seems a useless one, however, and might better be replaced by a simpler conception that males and females occupy a variety of different positions at different times ranging across a continuum of masculinity and femininity. Discussion of "latent" heterosexuals, for example, is rarely heard. It is only when deviation becomes a public issue that we turn to such artificial distinctions as "latent" and "overt."

There are as many variations in homosexuality as there are in heterosexuality. Attempts to classify homosexual acts along the simple dimensions of active-passive or masculine-feminine ignore the fact that primary and secondary sexual roles may be as interchangeable in the relation of one male to another as in the relationship of a male to a female (Guttmacher, 1961). Some persons can casually enjoy both homosexual and heterosexual acts or will indulge in transitory homosexuality when women are not accessible, yet consider their basic orientation to be heterosexual. While an individual may regularly prefer one form of gratification to all others, it is not unusual for him temporarily to shift roles with partners of either sex.

It is also true that only a limited number of male homosexuals can be identified by the mythical overt predominance of feminine mannerisms, affectations, or dress (Bergler, 1956; Karpman, 1954). Some effeminate men shun homosexual activity at the same moment that their seemingly masculine counterparts are its most avid seekers. Some homosexuals are hustlers who openly prostitute themselves (Ginsburg, 1967), and some homosexuals are bisexual with predominantly heterosexual contact coupled with homosexual encounter of an episodic, secret, or impulsive sort in response to stress or intoxication during which restraints and inhibitions are lowered. Among those for whom a member of the same sex is the greatest attraction, sexual gratification can come from rectal intercourse, oral-genital relations, or masturbation by another (Hooker, 1957).

According to Bieber (1967), the sex life of homosexuals differs from that of heterosexuals in that "homosexuals are more preoccupied with sex than are heterosexuals; they begin sexual practices earlier, and are more often sexually active in pre-adolescence, adolescence, and adulthood" (p. 965). In Bieber's study of homosexuals, "35 percent of the sample were already aware of their sexual interest in males by the time they were 10 years old; about 80 percent had this awareness by the age of 16; less than 10 percent became aware of their inversion after the age of 20" (p. 965).

For each acknowledged sexual deviant there are untold numbers of persons who have homosexual fantasies and impulses yet manage to control their outward behavior and make a socially acceptable adjustment (Halleck, 1967). Some who find direct outlets for homosexual urges do so without public knowledge. Others engage in a flamboyant display that almost certainly assures their apprehension and punishment by society. Surprisingly, few sex offenses, of any kind, reported to the police lead to convictions in court and even fewer offenders are sent to jail (Dunham, 1951). In most cases, the convicted offender is a young, unmarried male with a police record (Pacht, Halleck, and Ehrmann, 1962).

The Sources of Homosexuality

Psychoanalytic theory relies heavily on the conclusion that "castration-anxiety" is fundamental to homosexuality. According to analytic theorists, the child equates his sexual apparatus with the measure of himself as a person and views the penis as a symbol of strength, masculinity, and power. Threatened by the fantasied possibility that he may suffer amputation of his penis by an angry father figure and so lose the qualities of strength and power essential to successful living, the child deviates sexually in an unconscious attempt to ward-off such an evil fate and to maintain an intact self-image. The child's concern about his penis is reflected in his anxious concern about the presence or absence of this organ in other males and in the female. As Friedman (1959) noted, "while the fetishist and the transvestite . . . deny that the female lacks a penis, the homosexual accepts this fact but feels threatened by it" (p. 595).

In many instances the male homosexual "acts out" fantasy solutions to his masculine-feminine identity problems by becoming, in relationship to other males, the kind of child that would be most acceptable to the father whom he could never quite please or satisfy. Thus, the maturing male can assume the female role as a means of becoming "like" the mother in order, in fantasy, to be attractive to a rejecting father. Contact with strong, powerful males at a sexual level may be the unconsciously fantasied means of gaining worth and power by association.

In the studies of East (1946) and Bieber (1962), homosexuals were reported to have experienced seduction early in their youth (often before 14 years of age). While this event in itself is considered insufficient to produce lifelong patterns of homosexuality, it is the kind of experience that could easily fit the emotional needs of a youngster whose family pattern is already pathogenic.

The case of Matt T. illustrates one path of development of the homosexual.

MATT T.

The evolution of Matt's homosexuality to this final sad state of affairs was unspectacular and subtle. As a child he had always been very neat and clean, and he had preferred the company of girls in his neighborhood because all the boys were rough and dirty. His mother made him stay away from some of the tougher boys near his home and, after awhile, he felt about them the way his mother did. This preference for the company of females had a firm basis in his experience. Matt was a frail and a pretty child much admired by a covey of doting aunts who rewarded both his natural good looks and his girl-like behavior. His male cousins, envious at how admired he was by adults, looked forward to the signal that it was time for the children to go out and play together while the elders talked. This moment would produce a sinking feeling in Matt since he knew the outcome of this play would be physical and emotional torture for him at the hands of his revenge-seeking male relatives.

Boys knew almost instinctively that he was a sissy who would not fight back. In any group of young children, there are always girls who have begun to evaluate the attractiveness of males according to their toughness, fearlessness, bravado, and physical skill. Matt became a point-getter for some adventurous, fearless, and girl-conscious boys. These boys knew that by abusing Matt they enhanced their own status in the eyes of girls at the same time that they nourished their own underfed ego. With each punishment visited on him by other boys, Matt drifted further and further from the feeling that he was one of them.

By adolescence, Matt's attitudes, interests, skills, and patterns of behavior leaned more to the feminine than the masculine side. His status as a social boy-girl was joked about in high school and he, along with the others, came to admire the swashbuckling, all-American male heroes each school has. Matt hoped desperately one of them would notice him and include him in the inner circle of those who were admired and imitated. Matt tried to be "one of the boys" but he could never carry it off very convincingly. Matt double dated, for example, with other couples. At these times he engaged in a painful charade of pretense about his masculinity. He treated everything with innuendo and double meaning and played the part of a young and vigorous sex maniac. In the back seat of a car, he acted out the part of a leering, sneering romeo who was not to be denied by the innocence of his date. Matt's painful and inept attempts to press home his demands met with a predictable fate: girls laughed, boys laughed, Matt was systematically tortured by all his so-called friends (McNeil, 1967; pp. 110–11).

In the Judeo-Christian view of man that dominates our society, reproduction is the primary aim of sexual activity. This outlook inevitably has caused a limitation of freedom in heterosexual impulse expression and a stern rejection of homosexuality as perverse and sinful. In fact, the modern term sodomy (anal intercourse) had its origin in the practice of pederasty (anal intercourse with a boy or young man) reported in the biblical cities of Sodom and Gommorah. The Christian Reformation did little to extend or modify our moral beliefs about sexuality.

It was in the late 1800's that homosexuality became an issue of psychiatric concern. It must be recalled that when psychiatry first took note of homosexuality it was considered a form of degeneracy based on hereditary taint—a constitutional event for which little remedy was possible beyond exhorting the patient to exercise willpower. The then existing views of homosexuality looked not only to genetic predisposition as an explanation but added accidental exposure to homosexual assault in childhood, physical third sexedness (biological imperfections), and need for variety of sexual experience as other relevant possibilities. It was Freud's (1938) insight into the complexity of sexual development that stimulated theorists to consider new and quite different views of sexuality free of genetic bias or accidents of fate.

Opler (1967) suggested, however, that Freud's theoretical account of homosexuality should be considered as merely one of many possible outcomes of sexual development peculiar to members of middle-class Viennese society. In Opler's experience, a host of other roles were possible for homosexuals in other societies and at other times in history. Homosexuality is prevalent in some cultures and absent in others; in some it is sanctioned and in others it is forbidden. Surveys of sexual life in various cultures underscore the complexity of the cultural learnings which, in some societies, dictates that virtually all males will engage in homosexual practices at some time in their lives (Ford and Beach, 1951). In other cultures, it is a rare phenomenon. Historically, the number of societies that have lent full and unqualified sanction to homosexuality is very limited indeed. Heterosexuality has been, and remains, the norm for human sexual experience.

While homosexuality may be an almost invisible social problem to the average individual, it is a primary source of difficulty in situations in which males are confined together without access to females. Every prison official, for example, must decide about the permissible sexual life of the inmates for whom he is responsible. The issue of sex in prisons is complicated by the fact that the possibilities of homosexual seduction and rape are compounded by all the usual difficulties of jealousy and fighting for sole possession of sexual objects as well as the personal and social stress of anti-homosexual feelings on the part of heterosexual prisoners.

As Oliver and Mosher (1968) report, "The aggressive homosexuals —referred to as 'wolves,' 'daddies,' or 'studs'—fight among themselves for access to the weak, submissive, and passive males—referred to as 'sweet boys'" (p. 323). Between the "sweet boys" and the "wolves," prison officials indicate that nearly 15 percent of the inmates are actively engaged in homosexual relations. This is undoubtedly a conservative estimate.

Oliver and Mosher (1968) studied a prison population of 25 heterosexuals, 25 homosexual insertees (those using some orifice of their body as a receptacle for the other's penis), and 25 homosexual insertors (those inserting their penis into some orifice of another male). An analysis of psychological test findings on these prisoners suggests that while the psychological adjustment of heterosexual prisoners was typical for persons with behavioral disorders (those prone to impulsive antisocial behavior and seeking excitement), such prisoners are fairly free of crippling anxiety.

For the homosexual insertees and insertors, the findings were different from those for the persons judged to be heterosexual. Interestingly, the homosexual insertors freely admitted to their deviant thoughts, feelings, and behaviors and were rebellious nonconformists, i.e., were openly accepting of a higher degree of psychopathology than were the heterosexual or homosexual insertee groups. In contrast, the insertees (when compared with heterosexuals) displayed much greater confusion about both personal and sexual identity and were more inhibited about expressing aggressive impulses.

These recent findings suggest one certain conclusion. We have yet to complete our explorations of hetero- and homosexuality—it is a complex situation. We are not certain if there is a personality form that is characteristic of individuals who play different parts in the homosexual as opposed to the heterosexual act. We know that different sexual roles demand different kinds and qualities of personal adjustment. We have yet to detect the exact nature of these differences or track back to their origin.

Biologists have not neglected consideration of homosexual phenomena. Friedman (1959), for example, reports the results of Steinbach's experiments, completed as early as 1912 and 1913, in which the glands of the opposite sex were grafted onto castrated animals. Following these grafts, the animals showed behavior appropriate to the opposite sex. It was this glandular-biological argument that fueled the fire of controversy about homosexuality and inheritance. Freud (1959) believed that while he could detail the psychic mechanisms of homosexuality, only biologists could uncover the ultimate physical basis of its occurrence. Psychogenic events are predominant in Freudian theory but he always allowed theoretical room for a collaborative biological underpinning.

There is no reliable body of data that conclusively indicates a biological, constitutional, or endocrinological basis for bisexuality or homosexuality. A child is born "polymorph perverse," to use Freud's term, and seeks gratification without regard for the mode or object of that gratification. As the child develops he learns the socially approved limits of sexual expression just as he learns of the cultural ideal for male and female sex roles. Interference in learning these roles may, of course, be fostered by distortions of body build or glandular functioning, but these events contribute only indirectly to a homosexual orientation to life. Biological "programming" of the individual who becomes homosexual is a convenient rationalization for this condition.

Lesbianism

Lesbianism has been carefully ignored by theorists (Heidensohn, 1968). It is not just that lesbians are thought to be fewer in number than male homosexuals, it is that throughout history females have been regarded as inferior to the male and their sexual activities of much less concern. Too, female homosexuals are less visible, less aggressive in seeking sexual partners, less often social problems, and their deviant adjustment more easily disguised even in the married state (Simon and Gagnon, 1967).

Among lesbians, one partner may take the masculine and the other partner the feminine role in an imitation of the husband-wife role and/or the mother-daughter relationship. The obsessive concern of the male homosexual in seeking a partner with a large penis is matched by the high value lesbians place on large, well-formed breasts. According to Bieber (1967) "homosexuals of both sexes seek to repair their damaged sexual functioning by attempts at achieving a magical unity with prominant symbols of masculinity and feminity—the penis and the breast" (p. 974). Female homosexuals are likely to establish longer-lasting liaisons with their partners than do their deviant male counterparts. But, the id relationship remains fixated at an adolescent level of emotional involvement and, as with male homosexuals, is subject to all the petty bickerings and jealousies of immature human beings.

Female homosexuals are thought to undergo a learning experience that differs from that of male homosexuals. Initially closely attached to the mother (as is the boy), the girl must achieve womanhood by abandoning her first love object and substituting a male for the mother. In contrast, the heterosexual male need only substitute another woman for the mother who is a primary love object in order to achieve a socially acceptable role. The lesbian may fail to achieve heterosexuality in one of two ways: (1) failure to substitute a male for the original female love object or (2) anxiety in the encounter with adult males and regression to a sexual object appropriate only for very young children.

Psychoanalytic theory suggests that homosexuals are made anxious by an undeniable awareness of their genitalia, an awareness that is incontrovertible evidence of their true biological sex. The female, lacking male genitalia (and thus, in fantasy, having suffered castration), denies the truth of her situation by donning the clothing of the male and assuming masculine characteristics and mannerisms. This denial of femininity may not only satisfy unconscious needs but act to ward off males who might otherwise make sexual advances to her. Not all lesbians appear masculine, of course, or act out their sexual fantasies overtly; some lesbians mistrust males, prefer the company of females, and never become sexually involved with either.

Fetishism

When sexual excitement and gratification are produced regularly by stimuli from inanimate objects rather than people, it is called a fetish (Lorand and Schneer, 1967). The fetishist is usually a male who violates common mores of sexual practice both by selecting an inanimate object for his sexual attentions and by having his sexual aims fall short of heterosexual experience. The objects chosen as a fetish are most often artifacts related symbolically to conventional objects of affection (a woman's shoes, underclothing, hair clippings, etc.). But, there may be no direct connection between the two or only a highly indirect one. Thus, the fetish article may represent a part of the female anatomy or it may be symbolic of womanhood in general. And, the sexual fetish may be a way of expressing deep, underlying hostility toward either specific frustrating love-objects or toward the female in general (Grant, 1953).

For a fetishist, the part stands for the whole—the object comes to represent or symbolize the person. Fur, for example, may be a representation of pubic hair and reflect an absorption or fascination with one part or aspect of normal sexual impulses. The object of the fetish may in itself induce orgasm or it may be only a part of the total stimulation that produces the full sexual experience.

The fetish may also mirror sado-masochistic needs; it may represent a humbling and derogation of the self as a necessary part of achieving orgasm in the sex act. Perhaps Lorand (1950) is correct when he suggests that fetishism keeps its victim from becoming homosexual at the same moment that it prevents him from becoming normal. Absorbed in representations and symbols of sexuality, the fetishist manages to avoid the direct heterosexual act. It is apparent that the sex life of the fetishist is heavily dependent on an active fantasy life and is limited most often to masturbation. Looking at photographs or drawings of impossibly heroically proportioned naked females would not fulfill the requirements of a fetish since, most often, the picture is a representation of and a temporary substitute for the real thing.

Pedophilia

It is the preference for children as sexual objects (pedophilia) that arouses the greatest concern in our culture (Halleck, 1965). Children are ideal sexual objects because they are much less threatening to the pedophile, less likely to reject him, and more easily influenced than adult sexual objects. Fear of adult sexuality may be part of the explanation for this kind of deviation but it is not a sufficient answer. The choice of biologically immature sexual objects, some theorists suspect, involves a neurotic acting out of unresolved childhood conflicts. For child molesters, the world of childhood is socially safer and sexually less anxiety producing. Since child victims of adult sexual attentions are most often related to, or friends of the attacker, there may also be a bond of affection and familiarity between them.

Revitch and Weiss's (1962) study of nearly 900 pedophiles in New Jersey confirms the report of Swenson and Grimes (1958) that violence (threats or force) is frequently used and the crime often committed under the influence of alcohol. Alcohol reduces the inhibitions of the pedophile, and as the opportunity for sexual contact with a child presents itself restraint disappears and molestation occurs.

Most pedophiles are partly or fully impotent and are able to give themselves pleasure only through fondling, exhibitionistic, or masturbatory activities. The pedophile is an inadequate personality in a variety of respects not the least of which is sexual; he is particularly incapable of managing adult heterosexual relationships (Mohr, Turner, and Jerry, 1964). Our society has powerful taboos against sexual practices involving children, and the repugnance of members of society toward those who practice pedophilia is intense. Such persons are regularly rejected by "normal" citizens and mistreated even by their fellow prisoners once they are jailed.

Deviant Sexual Modes

The method of achieving sexual gratification—i.e., the mode of its expression—is considered deviant when it is focused on other than heterosexual intercourse. Any of a variety or combination of modes of sexual expression may be an integral part of the heterosexual experience and still be considered within the normal range, but when these "part expressions" of sexuality become exclusively the total sexual experience, we treat the behavior as pathological.

Masturbation, for example, is sex without a partner (except in fantasy) and could not be considered a model form of adult sexuality (Evans, 1968). Masturbation, despite the fact that it is universally practiced by young males and by adults for whom no sexual object is available, has always been viewed with suspicion in our society (Masters, 1967). In earlier days a variety of nervous disorders and physical disabilities were attributed to "excessive" masturbation, but much of this attitude has disappeared along with the many old wives' tales calculated to reinforce concensus in sexual practices. As recently as 1914, the United States Children's Bureau publication *Infant Care* told parents that masturbation was harmful and could easily get out of control. Anxiety about masturbation is occasioned both by conflict about accepting the growing sexuality of the child and the desire to deny it by thinking the child is "too young" for such behavior. Modern views of masturbation are much less restrictive.

Any sexual experience that is limited exclusively to oral-genital, anal-genital, or masturbatory contact is considered deviant since it falls short of total involvement in the heterosexual act. By the same standards of measurement, orgasm that cannot be accomplished without sadistic, masochistic, exhibitionistic, or voyeuristic behavior is deviant. Again, each of these tendencies is judged to be normal if it is not exaggerated by being excessively intense or the sole means to orgasm. It is obviously difficult to judge how much is "too" much.

Voyeurism

Before beginning a description of voyeurism we must pause just long enough to reassure the reader that if visual enjoyment of the naked body is to be considered an emotional disorder, then the great majority of the members of our society must be described in pathological terms. Ideally, each society should evolve to that state of psychological maturity in which the body is accorded exactly that degree of interest and enthusiasm it deserves as an ordinary part of human existence. Unfortunately, most modern societies have fallen far short of the ideal hoped for. As a consequence, viewing the naked body can be a sexually deviant practice for some persons; for the majority of us it is a gratifying, stimulating experience that is an integral part of heterosexual expression.

When looking at undressed sexual objects is the primary source of sexual excitement and when such looking takes the place of sexual intercourse, we label it voyeurism. The true voyeur achieves sexual excitement most often when he (and it is most often a he) is able to spy, secretly, on the undressed female. It is the sadistic aspect of this action (taking what she would not give freely) that produces sexual excitement, and this is often coupled with the excitement of risk of discovery.

Voyeurism among male children is a reasonably normal stage in the progression from infantile to adult sexuality. For the budding male such activity has as its aim unravelling the mysteries of sex and establishing, in fantasy, the role he will one day play in adult sexual affairs. In societies less restricted sexually, the frequency of voyeurism is greatly reduced. Our society does, of course, provide some outlets for the voyeuristic impulse—burlesque shows, topless waitresses, mini-skirts, and "girlie" magazines—but these outlets are officially permitted, culturally sanctioned, and without the element of risk and illicitness occasioned by stealing a view of what you would not otherwise be privileged to see.

The adult voyeur gets gratification by watching intercourse between other people and has a much more complicated set of dynamics. His sexual excitement may be occasioned more by the view of male genitalia and male sexual activity than by witnessing sexual expression in the female. The voyeur fears women. The excitement he feels when spying on them when they are naked and unsuspecting reassures him that he is indeed more cunning than most as well as capable of sexual response even if it is an excited, tension-laden, heart-pounding orgasm experienced alone and secretly. The greatest threat to the voyeur would be if the victim of his spying were to detect him and invite him to heterosexual encounter. The voyeur (the Peeping Tom of popular literature) is a passive, rarely dangerous person.

Exhibitionism

For the male, exhibiting his penis to females and masturbating when he has their attention has been interpreted as a symptom of the need not only to reassure himself of his maleness, i.e., that he has a penis, but to convince himself that this organ is powerful, potent, and impressive to the female. The fate worse than death for an exhibitionist must be to be laughed at and ridiculed during his exhibition or, worse yet, to be ignored completely. In periods of mounting anxiety, the exhibitionist must show his penis to reinforce his judgment of his worth as a human being by observing fear and shock at such a masterful display. Most often exhibitionists use young children as an audience.

Exhibitionistic acts were described, long ago, as instantaneous and compulsive outbursts, and this inability to resist an impulse remains characteristic of the exhibitionist today. The male exhibitionist shows his genitalia to strangers in an aggressive act that intrudes on their privacy. And this is related dynamically to the apparent natural exhibitionism of young male children. The male exhibitionist engages in behavior that reassures him of what less troubled males take for granted—masculinity (Blane and Roth, 1967; Christoffel, 1956). The exhibitionist feels deeply guilty about his compulsion to make a public display of the anxiety that is so basic to his makeup. Interestingly, exhibitionists will "squeal" on one another to the police—no doubt out of fear of being upstaged by other exhibitionists. As Ellis (1942) has noted, the exhibitionist seems to over-evaluate the worth and meaning of his penis in an attempt to deny the truth that he cannot face—that he is not a man.

The degree of pathology detected among exhibitionists is unusually high. Henninger (1941) analyzed 51 cases of indecent exposure and found 14 would have been classified as emotionally immature, 10 mentally retarded, 8 psychotic, and 4 chronic alcoholics. Mohr, Turner, and Jerry (1964) indicate that, in some instances, exhibitionism precedes the act of child molesting. They state that almost all of the young adults apprehended for exhibitionism were married before exhibitionism became a part of overt behavior. These quiet, unassuming, immature men responded to sexual deprivation or marital conflict by being unable to resist the overwhelming urge to display their genitals in public.

Theorists have treated male exhibitionists with hypnosis (Ritchie, 1968) and out-patient group therapy (Witzig, 1968). They consider exhibitionism a form of obsessive-compulsive sexual disorder that differs little, dynamically, from neurotic disorders that have settled on other than sexual modes and objects as outlets. At best, exhibitionism is ·a minor social problem, since its frequency is rare and its practice is only modestly offensive.

Transvestism

The urge to dress in the clothes of members of the opposite sex (transvestism) is almost exclusively a male preoccupation. The transvestite may become extremely adept at playing the role of the female, and in full disguise he acts out a fantasy of the feminine part of himself. Fearing women, he can, by becoming one in appearance, be his "own" woman —acting and responding in ways he alone dictates. He tames his fears by playing them out in a controlled situation.

Cross-dressing is a way of expressing male comfort as a female and the unconscious wishes to be one. In addition, an important part of the sexual aspect of this experience is genital contact with the silk-like textures of female garments. This in itself is sufficient to provide sexual gratification for some transvestites (Lukianowicz, 1960).

Interestingly, women frequently dress transsexually without evoking comment in our culture. The absence of social reaction to the adoption of masculine-like attire by females is, in part, reflective of our social disconcern with females and, in part, because the essence of being feminine is often retained to offset the apparel. A male transvestite with a full grown beard would be as unconvincing as a female sex symbol clad in skin tight slacks.

The psychoanalytic view of transvestism suggests that the transvestite (who most often is not an active homosexual) unconsciously believes females once had a penis but lost it via castration. Fearing the same fate, the transvestite dresses like a woman and "pretends" that women are not castrated, i.e., he is a woman who still has a penis hidden by clothes. Dressed like a woman, the male can assume all the passive-receptive characteristics of the female while he retreats from the anxiety-producing male role (Nielson, 1960). Among transvestites, as well as homosexuals, the riddle of male-female identity never gets solved in a socially acceptable manner. It is a riddle complicated by unresolved conflict about mothers, fathers, males, and females.

Transvestites and fetishists make similar use of feminine clothing for sexual stimulation and as sexual objects. But, as Friedman (1959) indicates, "unlike the fetishist, the transvestite is not 'in love' with a specific article, as such, but utilizes articles of apparel of the opposite sex as a means of attaining orgasm and of facilitating identification with the other sex" (p. 599).

For some transvestites, wearing transsexual clothing is a first step in the fantasy-hope that surgical procedures can one day remove the last vestiges of biological sex identity. It is hoped surgical alteration of the sexual apparatus coupled with hormone treatment will transform the transvestite into a closer approximation of the preferred primary and secondary sexual characteristics. Dynamically, transvestities may be a complicated mixture of exhibitionist, fetishist, and homosexual. Surgical alteration of the body may add to rather than relieve the problem since it deals with such limited aspects of sex role, identity, and gender.

Sadism and Masochism

Sadism and masochism are terms derived from the works of the Marquis de Sade (1740–1814) and Leopold von Sachermasoch (1863–1895) who wrote extensively of their personal fantasies of sex coupled with pain, abuse, and humiliation. When inflicting physical or psychological pain on others is necessary for sexual excitement and pleasure, it is called sadism. When sexual excitement and gratification are possible only when one is being hurt or humiliated, it is called masochism. These conditions have been described by Freud (1938) as a fusion of sexual and aggressive impulses coupled with a distortion of the two in ways that seem deviant to the average citizen in our society. Since this intermixture of sex and aggression varies from time to time within the person, the condition might best be described as sadomasochism.

Sadomasochistic aspects of sexual experience are not always part of a consciously deviate pattern of interpersonal relations. The male who achieves his greatest sexual gratification with a male or female he can "use," humiliate, or abuse, or the person whose sexual satisfaction is best achieved when subject to this rough treatment may well be unaware that this pattern is an essential part of his personality. The male who whips or beats his sexual partner may be acting out a fantasy of destroying or rendering harmless the other person in order to feel safe relating sexually. Intercourse in such circumstances then becomes a form of rape-with-permission following the sadistic assault.

Males tend normally to be more aggressive in sexual relationships, and "rough" treatment of the others may, as an expression of male dominance and power, heighten the sexual experience. Sadism and sex mixed in their most extreme form produce a mode of gratification characteristic of persons who enjoy sex only when it is forced on others, i.e., sexual assault and rape. The sadist seeks out the masochist for their mutual sexual gratification. When sadistic or masochistic behavior is the only means to sexual gratification, or when it becomes extreme and intense, the probability is high that we are dealing with a psychotic rather than neurotic phenomenon.

THE TREATMENT OF
SEXUAL DEVIATION

One vexing problem in doing research on homosexuality and its many variants is the difficulty of gaining access to homosexual groups that have made some viable adjustment to this socially tabooed behavior. Homosexuals with severe personality disorders, homosexuals sufficiently anxious to seek psychotherapy, or homosexuals entangled with the law, all form special cases that may not be truly representative of the larger population of homosexuals. Hooker (1963) reported that it took as long as five years to arrange some interviews with homosexuals for whom exposure would mean social catastrophe or discharge from the armed forces (Doidge and Holtzman, 1960). Our system of laws still views homosexuality as a crime (Wolfenden Report, 1963) and, most often, our society imprisons sex deviates to keep them from violating the mores of our society (East, 1946).

Bieber (1962) reported that in psychoanalytic treatment only 2 of 28 patients changed to heterosexuality after fewer than 150 hours of therapeutic contact and the rate was little improved in those who experienced between 150 and 350 hours of psychoanalysis. In the latter case, only 9 of 40 patients switched. Group therapy within the confines of an institution has been attempted, but the results have not been very reassuring (Cabeen and Coleman, 1961).

A recent attempt to change the perverse response into a "normal" one has involved conditioning and learning techniques (McGuire, Carlisle, and Young, 1965) in which the stimulus, i.e., a naked male, that evokes a socially unacceptable sexual response is paired with a painful or noxious stimulus (electric shock) to "condition" withdrawal or revulsion when the deviant sexual object appears. Learning theory is used to explain the acquisition of normal and deviant responses and "unlearning" through conditioning used as a solution.

A wide range of treatments has been attempted with little success. Drugs, electric shock, castration, and hormone administration have all shown an initial promise that has yet to bear fruit. When the literature of homosexuality is reviewed (Miller, Bradley, Gross, and Wood, 1968) and the varieties of treatment recorded, it is apparent that no possibility has gone unexplored. Most recently learning theory (Wickramasekera, 1968), behavior therapy (Ramsay and van Velzen, 1968), aversion therapy (Marks, 1968), and LSD (Martin, 1967) have been tried.

Yet, clinicians and researchers are actively engaged in the search for new answers to treatment and for new means of diagnosing and detecting the sex deviates in our society (Davids, Joelson, McArthur, 1956; Friberg, 1967; Hooker, 1958; Kopp, 1962; Lanyon, 1967; Panton, 1960). It is doubtful that any simple solution to these problems will be discovered. The problem has been studied again and again by groups formed to examine these continuing issues (Glueck, 1956) and textbooks and encyclopedias exploring sex problems continue to detail the dimensions of the problem of homosexuality (Allen, 1962; Ellis and Abarnel, 1961; Wahl, 1967). To date, our progress has been less than spectacular.

It remains true that the most positive approaches to homosexuality rely on effective early detection and prevention. Since pre-homosexual children exhibit symptoms early in life, it would seem reasonable to assume that some form of public education might make this problem less critical in our society. Psychotherapeutic intervention early in the life of the child may be vital in altering these patterns of behavior before they become a fixed way of life.

SUMMARY

Sexual deviation constitutes a serious social problem in our culture despite the relative infrequency of its occurrence. The forms of sexual deviation include unusual intensity and frequency of sexual activity (impotence, frigidity, nymphomania, satyriasis, and promiscuity), unacceptable modes of sexual expression (sadism, masochism, voyeurism, transvestism, exhibitionism, masturbation, and oral-genital and anal-genital contact), and choice of deviant sexual objects (homosexuality, lesbianism, incest, bestiality, fetishism, and pedophilia).

Theoretical explanations of sexual deviation are varied, but a primary focus has been on confusion and conflict in learning what society defines as a proper sexual role, i.e., the acquisition of a sexual identity that matches one's biological inheritance. Clinical studies have dispelled many of the myths and romantic fictions with regard to sexual deviation and sexual deviants by indicating that the sexual deviant hardly presents a heroic image in real life. The deviant is usually immature, anxious, self-centered, and inadequate as a human being. He seems fixated at a level of development in which he repeats over and over an inappropriate and inadequate solution to a vital aspect of relating to others.

The demands of the male role to achieve, accomplish, compete, perform, be assertive, aggressive, commanding, and decisive prove to be impossible for about 4 percent of the males in our population, and they seek refuge by denying the essential facts of life—assuming the less demanding female role allows them to be passive and cared for rather than actively caring for others.

Sexual deviation is threatening to those who consider themselves normal. Our social response has most often been anxious, primitive, and punitive. When therapy has been applied to cases of adult sexual deviation the results have been unimpressive. Sexual deviations seem to be formed early in life and highly resistive to change in later years. Our therapeutive methods most often succeed in those instances in which the victim is highly motivated for treatment and anxious about his condition. New approaches seem to hold promise, but this may be an unwarranted optimism.

The Addictions 10

America has been described as a nation of addicts—a society heavily dependent on alcohol, tranquilizers, sedatives, energizers, narcotics, caffeine, nicotine, aspirin, marijuana, psychedelic consciousness expanders, and patent medicines. It is a severe and undoubtedly exaggerated indictment of our culture but we must be aware that our addictions are indeed many and varied. And, in terms of sheer numbers and human misery, the abuse of alcohol certainly heads the list.

ALCOHOLISM

In the book *The Billion Dollar Hangover* (Coppolino and Coppolino, 1965) it is estimated that at least 800,000 problem drinkers (persons for whom alcohol causes occasional problems) are employed in agricultural and industrial enterprises in America. The problem drinker, or his more intensely involved counterpart, the alcoholic, is a chronic problem since he has a high rate of absenteeism, twice the accident rate of his co-workers, and a life span shorter by twelve years than that of his fellow worker. Forty million work days a year are said to be lost to our collossal national hangover, and it is impossible to estimate how many mistake-laden, error-strewn, inefficient work hours go undetected.

The formula for an alcoholic can be presented simply and directly (Coppolino and Coppolino, 1965):

1. He says, "I can take it or leave it alone," but he can't.
2. He alibis saying, "I'm expected to drink in my line of work."

129

3. He takes a drink in the morning in order to be able to get to the job in reasonable shape.
4. He senses trouble ahead and switches briefly to less potent liquids.
5. He becomes antisocial and ends up drinking alone.
6. He stays away from his job and avoids his ex-friends and former loved-ones.

At least one-half of the "accidental" deaths in traffic are thought to be caused by drinking drivers and alcohol is a vital factor in homicide and suicide in our society; one sure way of being a "successful" suicide is to drink heavily before you make an attempt on your life (Laughlin, 1967). The person bent on suicide may drink until he produces a chemical euphoria that helps him deny that he is depressed. But, when he sobers up, he may be overwhelmed by the massive depression he temporarily dulled with alcoholic stupor.

Drinking to excess can also be described in geographic terms; the citizens of California rank highest with those in New Jersey, New Hampshire, and New York close behind. These alcoholics are not the popularized denizens of the Skid Rows of our nation. They are the respectable citizens who are your neighbors. The extent of individual human misery attendant on what some define as problem drinking is difficult to comprehend, and if the individual's distress is multiplied by a factor of 5, 10, or 20 (wife, children, relatives, friends, employers, etc.), it becomes an enormous public health problem.

Stages and Types of Alcoholism

In small amounts, alcohol is a drug which depresses those parts of the brain that usually inhibit the raw expression of impulses, needs, and anxieties seldom apparent in a sober state (Conger, 1951, 1956). Up to a point alcohol facilitates social interaction by making us less anxious; after that point, it disorders sensation, perception, and behavior and produces negative social consequences. Consequently, alcohol is popularly thought to be a stimulant since behavior following drinking is more boisterous and uninhibited than usual. Actually, alcohol stimulates uninhibited behavior by depressing the "higher" brain centers, i.e., those most recently acquired in man's evolutionary history, those that normally exert social control.

As the concentration of alcohol in the blood increases, there is a matched diminution of intellectual, sensory, perceptual, and refined muscular functioning. The initial sharpening of perceptual and sensory experience while drinking is soon followed by a progressive decline (Chafetz, 1967); how rapid and destructive this decline will be depends on the amount of alcohol consumed during a particular period of time.

Behavior changes occur in direct relation to the rate at which alcohol is fed into the blood stream through the stomach and gastrointestinal tract. The rate of absorption, of course, depends on a variety of factors such as size of the person, his rate of metabolic activity, and the food contained in the stomach. (A stomach full of mashed potatoes can absorb alcohol and slow the rate of its entry into the blood stream.) In yet unmeasured ways psychological factors such as mood, emotional state, and the surroundings in which drinking takes place seem to affect the response to alcohol (Mayfield and Allen, 1967). Simply put, you can get drunk quicker at a victory celebration than you can at a wake.

Theoretical stages and types of alcoholism are described by Jellinek (1952, 1960). A developing alcoholic begins with a symptomatic *pre-alcoholic* phase in which he discovers liquor provides an escape from crisis; it reduces tension and bolsters self-confidence. In the *prodromal* phase that follows the victim drinks heavily, furtively, suffers blackouts, and what was once a social beverage becomes a drug. In the next, or *crucial,* phase of his drinking habits he begins to drink until he can't absorb any more, loses control over his behavior, and is unable to decide whether he will continue to drink. The social and personal deterioration appears first in the crucial phase when he engages in drinking "benders" that last for days or weeks, starts to experience symptoms of "withdrawal" when without liquor, begins drinking early in the morning to regain the psychological balance needed to face the demands of the day ahead, and displays a grossly impaired efficiency in his work.

As the compulsive drinking escalates, he becomes the not very pretty picture of a common drunk (Freedman and Wilson, 1967). He drinks nearly continuously, suffers physically and psychologically from too much liquor and not enough food, is unresponsive to the distress evident among those close to him, and is desperate in his quest to remain blissfully drugged to the pain and anxiety of life. Not all alcoholics suffer exactly the same set of symptoms, of course, since not all alcoholics are precisely alike in personality and temperament. Jellinek, divides drinkers into Alpha, Beta, Gamma, and Delta types, for example. These types range not only from least to most severe in degree of alcoholism but each type is characterized by different needs for, and responses to, alcohol.

The Alpha alcoholic, for example, uses alcohol to relieve tension and, in the process, violates the social rules of when, where, and how much one should drink. But the Alpha alcoholic can abstain from drinking completely when it is crucial to do so and he can control the amount he drinks. The Alpha drinker may maintain this condition throughout his lifetime without progressing to more frequent drinking. In contrast, the most severe alcoholic, the Delta, acquires an increased tolerance for alcohol (he has to drink more to get high), his body gets accustomed to alcoholic saturation, and he needs alcohol to feel normal. Unfortunately, he cannot abstain from drinking and he suffers withdrawal symptoms when deprived of the drug. The Alpha pattern is one of psychological dependence on alcohol; the Delta pattern describes a full blown physiological as well as psychological dependence.

The case of Nick L. relates vividly some of the difficulties posed for and by an alcoholic in our society.

NICK L.

When the drinks came Nick's eyes lighted up, he grinned, and rubbed his hands together in high glee. He downed the martini in one gulp and with a smooth, uninterrupted movement raised his eyes to establish the whereabouts of the waitress and lifted his empty glass to signal his needy condition.

For a moment it was as though I had disappeared and he sat alone at the table. All of his attention was focused on restoring his glass to its previous state of fullness. That done, he suddenly realized that I had not yet touched my drink. Nick pointed to it, smiled broadly, and observed that there was no such thing as a strong martini, only weak people. I used this opening to move in on the issue that had brought me to the bar in the first place. . . .

Nick was always less than the dominant, aggressive, assertive, decisive male he fancied himself to be. He devoted more than the usual amount of time to cocktail conversation of the "I really told him off" variety. When he did take issue with someone's view of the world, he was careful to hobble each hostile word with apologetic modifiers led by a smile that pleaded for acceptance. Nick hated disagreement of any sort almost as much as he hated to say no to anyone. Nick could only be comfortable saying no if he functioned exclusively as an innocent messenger bearing ill tidings. Even then it would cross his mind that kings once executed those bearing bad news. . . .

Nick's hangovers were spectacular. As he said, the first sensation is blinding pain. It's like what I imagine a brain tumor would feel like. Your head hurts so bad that you cannot even open your eyes. I go to the bathroom and swallow some aspirin but they always make me throw up. I go back to bed and wait till I get sick then I rush to the john and have the "dry heaves" for nearly an hour. My throat is raw for the whole next day and the first drink I take nearly kills me. Then I go back to sleep but I don't sleep long because I have nightmares and wake up dying of thirst. A Bloody Mary in the morning is the only solution. When I can get one I nearly choke on it, but in about five minutes my head comes back to my shoulders and my eyes start to focus again.

The hardest part about being drunk is that you have to pretend you aren't. Acting steady is difficult when everybody is staring at you. You have to watch not to fumble your money, or laugh too much, or do things you know you can't manage. I got so that I would hang around in bars where a lot of guys got crocked and nobody paid any attention to them. The trouble with those joints was that somebody always wanted to fight or some queer would sidle up to you and proposition you. Being steady in public was not nearly so hard as trying not to look drunk in front of your own kids. That was rough because I think they always knew something was wrong and that their daddy was "sick" again (McNeil, 1967; pp. 127, 128, 130).

Alcohol has always been a problematical part of human social existence since it is a drug widely used to relieve emotional tension yet available without medical prescription. Alcoholism has been viewed with a mixture of amusement and alarm over the course of history—affluent and "well-bred" alcoholics have always been tolerated in society with greater grace than their drunken, disheveled, brawling, lower-class counterparts. Rank has always had its privileges and freedom to overindulge in alcohol seems to be one of them (Alexander and Selesnick, 1965).

A great many intelligent and creative men have described alcohol as an aid to the creative process. Coppolino and Coppolino (1965), for example, mention the names of a number of able, intelligent, creative writers who fell victim to dependence on alcohol—Upton Sinclair, O. Henry, Brendan Behan, Stephen Crane, Dylan Thomas, F. Scott Fitzgerald, and Eugene O'Neill. The list of eminent persons in other walks of life who found solace in alcohol could be extended infinitely. As Menninger (1938) has suggested, the alcoholic of whatever creative bent may still be running from a nameless and unspeakable terror; the brightness of the creative alcoholic may appear early in life only to be drowned in alcohol as his conflicts catch up with him.

Little is known about the female alcoholic since she may resolve her problems by drinking to excess in the privacy of her own home (Curlee, 1967). But it is estimated there are nearly a million females who cannot exercise moderation with liquor. At the moment only one female for every five or six males has this problem, but the number of women alcoholics seems to be rising as they acquire equal status with the male in our society. The number of female "occasional" drinkers is equal to that of males (about 48 percent) but "heavy" drinking is primarily a male problem. Males who drink heavily are more likely than women to engage in behavior that will involve them with social agencies, hospitals, and police. Women, more often than men, drink just to the point of relief from anxiety without exceeding proper limits. They are, thus, less likely to come into conflict with society. Yet, the behavioral patterns of male and female alcoholics are quite similar, and both are likely to come from broken homes or homes in which parents had a drinking problem.

Theories of Alcoholism

Theoretical views about the causes of alcoholism have been many and varied but they do not yet add up to a comprehensive account of all the behavioral facts of drunkenness. Buss (1966) describes four theories of alcoholism worth recounting here—cultural, learning, dynamic, and biological.

Biological Theories

Biological theories have suggested physiological or endocrinological malfunction, nutritional deficiency, biochemical disorder, or brain pathology as possible sources of alcoholism. Unfortunately, the trustworthy empirical findings of these studies have been meager indeed. Less reliable scientific insight has emerged than free-wheeling speculation about possible biological determinants of who does or does not become the victim of the drug alcohol.

Biological theorists suggest, for example, that alcoholics may have inherited an inability to manufacture the basic enzymes needed to digest various foods. Thus, so goes the theory, the alcoholic craves those substances missing in his body and drinks to replenish them (Williams, 1947, 1959). This theory was greeted with enthusiasm at the time it was first proposed, but further research has cast considerable doubt on its accuracy (Lester and Greenberg, 1952).

Williams reached his conclusions by studying rats deprived of vitamins and then offered a choice of water or alcohol; the rats preferred alcohol. When offered a third choice (sugared water) in follow-up experiments, it became apparent that rats preferred this alternative to either alcohol or plain water. Failing to discover a biological basis for alcoholism in these experiments, researchers have since turned to exploring the different lengths of time it takes to reach the state of addictive alcoholism.

The Mayfield (1968A, 1968) experiments, for example, indicate that the emotional state of the heavy drinker is changed less by the ingestion of alcohol than the average person suspects. It may well be that the changes in mood caused by drinking are experienced most often by moderate rather than heavy drinkers. If so, we must revise some of our views of the emotional benefits obtained by heavy drinking.

Hope remains that refined and improved biochemical methods will one day produce more fruitful results, of course, but cultural and dynamic theories seem to offer a greater probability of scientific and theoretical breakthrough.

Cultural Theories

Cultural theorists point out that there seem to be clear-cut national and racial differences in rates of alcoholism and they look to family patterns in the culture for an explanation of the problem. In primitive societies the frequency of drunkenness and the general intake of intoxicating beverages seem related to the degree of anxiety the members of that culture experience attempting simply to survive, i.e., storms, possible crop failure, etc. (Horton, 1943).

In these circumstances alcohol washes away the sting of anxiety and becomes the drug most favored for escape from reality. Observations of the kind made by Horton must be tempered with healthy skepticism, however. We are not at all sure that drinking patterns in primitive cultures are not being overinterpreted or interpreted falsely when viewed through Western, technological, civilized eyes. The fact is that alcohol releases inhibitions and provides a marked short-term release for its consumers. Complicated theory with regard to storms and crops may be superfluous to our comprehension of primitives and alcohol.

In many countries alcohol (usually wine) is a food supplement used routinely with meals. Since patterns of alcoholism differ in whiskeydrinking as opposed to wine-drinking societies, cultural theorists feel social factors must be assessed if we are to understand alcoholism. Problem drinking happens also to be related to social class and ethnic background, i.e., the rate of alcoholism is higher among Irish than Americans and it is higher in the members of the middle than the lower classes (McCord, McCord, and Gudeman, 1959).

Sophisticated cultures form complicated rules about the use of alcohol ranging across total abstinence, ritual drinking, convivial drinking, or utilitarian drinking (Bales, 1946). The American society is a mixture of convivial (party-goers) and utilitarian (it's a part of the job) drinkers. The anxiety that impels us to drink is an interpersonal one forged in a competitive society.

Recent studies of drinking patterns among Negroes (Maddox, 1968) have indicated that we have long had a scientific blind spot for racial differences in use of alcohol. Limited available research suggests that middle-class Negroes almost universally use liquor as an outlet, are heavy drinkers (compared with white middle-class members), and frequently have social trouble connected with their drinking. The most interesting speculative observation suggests that Negro drinking patterns are those of "discomfort," i.e., a minority group member competing with a majority group in any culture will suffer strains and pressures for which alcohol can be a temporary remedy. In addition, heavy drinking can act to reinforce stereotypes held by members of the majority culture and can be a mixed act of defiance and self-destruction among Negro drinkers. Imagine how you might react to a lifetime of segregation, discrimination, and prejudice when the drug alcohol is easily available to ease the pain.

If you study the family structure in a culture, you must examine the wives of alcoholics to comprehend drunken behavior (Lernert, 1960).

These women (Whalen, 1953) tend to marry men who were already well on the road to alcoholism during the time of courtship and as the drinker moves deeper into his alcoholic haze, the wife rightfully, and perhaps with some pleasure and a sense of "I told you so," assumes a position as head of the household. Once firmly implanted in this position and adjusted to her new responsibilities, she may "hold court" for the sympathetic ministrations of others and may contribute to the drinker's difficulties by becoming a positive deterrent to well-meaning therapeutic attempts to teach her husband to walk without an alcoholic crutch.

Dynamic Theories

It is obvious that no single-factor, dynamic theory can account for the incredible complexity of the problem we have labeled alcoholism. It is not useful to dismiss this complicated issue by stating that excessive drinkers are "oral" or "passive-dependent" personalities (Fenichel, 1945). As Levy (1958) noted, alcohol may serve a variety of dynamic functions. Alcohol can, for example, be a legitimate excuse for the expression of impulses that would otherwise be forbidden in normal social congress. That is, a drinker can become hostile, abusive, and punishing of others but can deny responsibility for this behavior on the grounds that he was drunk at the time. Alcohol can dull the edge of severe anxiety, guilt, or blame or be used as a means of gratification in an otherwise cruel and unrewarding world.

There have been a great many attempts to pin down the dynamics of the alcoholic but these have most often been so broad, general, and unspecific that they seem equally descriptive of, and interchangeable with, a variety of other symptom pictures of any of a number of emotional disorders (Gomberg, 1968; Jones, 1968; Sanford, 1968). Personality factors dynamically predisposing to alcoholism may include early oral fixation (oral intake becomes a primary and continuing source of gratification), deep-seated fears of destruction by others (the victim drinks to dull the edge of the threat); or, a family constellation in which various combinations of a dominant, rejecting mother and a weak father (or the reverse—a severe father and an ineffectual mother) combine to produce an adult who may be impotent, hostile, frightened, or self-destructive. Such dynamic early encounters could result in alcoholism or as easily produce any of the species of neurotic patterns.

Given a distorted family situation in which he learns about himself and others, the growing child is forced to erect a number of psychological defenses against anxiety in an attempt to carve out a workable way of life. But, this statement is as true of other neurotic disabilities as it is of alcoholism. When these defenses prove inadequate to protect the alcoholic against an awareness of his personal shortcomings, he turns to heavy drinking as a means of easing his psychological pain just as other neurotics turn to other forms of self-destruction. Until the dynamics of alcoholism are differentiated from those of a variety of other neuroses and character disorders, we will make little progress in our efforts to detect potential alcoholism early in life and prescribe adequately for its treatment.

Researchers describe excessive drinkers as persons suffering personality or character disorders marked by hostile, depressed, dependent, and immature behavior (Zwerdling and Rosenbaum, 1959). The narcissistic, self-centered adult is described as easy prey for the devastating effects of alcohol.

One caution should be added. Without a much more elaborate and detailed account of current dynamic theories of alcoholism, there may be a great temptation to view progression to the alcoholic state as a fairly simple and direct series of steps. The truth is certainly far from being so simple; the alcoholic does not easily and passively slide into drunken oblivion, rather he fights, strives, regroups his defenses, attempts to reassemble himself into a better adjusted state, and suffers deeply from attacks of anxiety, guilt, and shame as he privately appraises his own behavior (Isbell, 1955; Menaker, 1967).

While alcoholism, as a symptom, can be a dynamic part of any of a great variety of disorders of living, studies suggest that alcoholics have a roughly common dynamic history:

1. AN INABILITY TO HANDLE TENSION IN A MATURE MANNER. He easily, and with little apparent cause, feels rejected by others, retreats from conflicts, avoids unpleasantness of any kind, vacillates in committing himself or making decisions, and cannot tolerate tension for long periods of time.

2. A DEEP DEPENDENCY ON OTHER PEOPLE. Finding that others seem more able, more capable, or stronger, alcoholics become passive and, much like a young child, seek to be cared for and protected by others. When thrust into situations that demand independence and performance, they retreat to alcohol to escape tension.

3. A SEVERE UNEXPRESSED HOSTILITY TO THOSE CLOSEST TO HIM. The need to be dependent on others provokes resentment and hostility that gets pushed out of consciousness only to appear in indirect and disguised ways. Consciously, the alcoholic insists he loves those who are closest to him; unconsciously, his behavior indicates the opposite is true.

4. EGOCENTRICITY IS A PART OF THE LEGACY OF HIS EARLY DEVELOP-
MENT. The immaturity of the alcoholic is most apparent in the degree to which he feels sorry for himself and feels people pick on him.
He acts like a jealous child who senses his brothers or sisters are
favored by the parents.

These factors are primarily psychological in nature and some theorists
suggest that they alone are not sufficient to produce alcoholism. These
theorists insist that something like a physiological "readiness" or "bodily
compliance" is needed to help the process on its way. Physiological
theories of alcoholism have suggested that repeated, severe alcoholic intoxication in the very young person (early drinker) produces brain
damage that renders the drinker less able to tolerate alcohol and leads
him to seek alcohol as an aid to adequate brain functioning.

Middle-of-the-road theorists have tried to bridge this gap by suggesting
that it takes both aspects of human makeup to produce a hopeless drunk
—psychological readiness and physiological vulnerability. Again, there is
little trustworthy experimental evidence to confirm or disprove this combined theoretical approach. This is a grossly oversimplified view of the
contribution of physiologists to our comprehension of the problem of
alcohol. Their hypotheses are much more refined than those reported
here, but the absence of experimental backing for such speculations pre-
cludes a more lengthy account.

It is easy, then, to agree with Chafetz (1967) who discards the notion
that a single personality configuration exists for alcoholism. Problems with
alcohol are known to occur in any and all types of psychological disorder
but psychological disorder is just one manifestation of a complicated and
complex set of pressures that lead the individual to choose this, rather
than an alternative, way to solve his problems. As Chafetz notes,
". . . study after study has shown that offspring drink like their parents:
heavy drinkers produce heavy drinking children, abstainers produce
abstainers, and moderate drinkers produce moderate drinkers" (p. 1013).
The exceptions to these rules are, perhaps, cases best explained in terms
of the psychodynamics of the individual.

Learning Theories

Learning theorists have approached the issue of alcoholism by referring
to how all other human responses are learned and become habitual
(Conger, 1951, 1956).

Storm and Smart (1965), for example, maintain that the drunken condition must be differentiated from the sober state to explain the apparent

differences between the person when sober and the same person when drunk. If you begin drinking when young and drink excessively, they believe you increase the possibility that you will learn one pattern of behavior while drinking and a distinctly different pattern when sober. Thus, telling a sober person to behave himself will have little effect if the sober and drunken states are experienced as disconnected, separate, unique, learned conditions. Storm and Smart go on to suggest that through a series of conditioned responses the first drink leads to the second, the second to the third, etc. The inability to break this chain of "drink = feel good = have another drink" marks the alcoholic. What the theory fails to explain is how some persons manage to drink without going out of control while others find alcohol an unmanageable drug.

There is no essential incompatibility between dynamic and learning theories. They both address themselves to the same process with dynamic theory describing the broad direction and outcome of development while learning theory focuses more closely on the step-by-step mechanics by which the end-product is attained. It is when learning theory becomes excessively mechanical and overconcerned with detail that conflict between the two viewpoints occurs.

The Treatment of Alcoholism

Treatment of alcoholism takes a variety of forms and has a series of aims (Rosen and Gregory, 1965). The first step, usually, is a drying-out process in which alcohol is withdrawn and suspected vitamin deficiencies are remedied. This may be coupled with the prescription of stimulants to restore the patient's metabolism to a more normal condition. The process of withdrawal from addiction to alcohol is not a pleasant event. Deprived of alcohol, the heavy drinker is exposed to a mixture of psychological and physiological experiences that may include an increase in blood pressure, pulse rate, body temperature, dehydration (dry mouth and skin), and pain. Psychologically, the drying-out alcoholic feels shaky, frightened, restless, depressed, and suffers insomnia (Godfrey, Kissin, and Downs, 1958; Isbell, 1955). While this drying out does not cure the alcoholic, it at least returns him to a state in which he can be treated.

As a next step he may be given chemicals that will induce nausea and vomiting if he drinks. Antabuse, for example, alters the patient's metabolism to produce violent illness if he drinks alcohol in the next several days. If the patient can be induced to continue taking Antabuse it is hoped he will eventually be able to avoid alcohol in any form at any time. Once released from the hospital, however, the determined alcoholic can simply cease taking his medication and return to his previous drinking habits (Quinn and Henbest, 1967). In some instances determined alcoholics have been reported to drink despite their nausea.

Attempts have been made to relieve alcoholism with LSD, tranquilizers, antidepressants, electroconvulsive therapy, and psychotherapy (Kurland, Unger, Shaffer, and Savage, 1967). The results have been less than satisfying. No drug has yet proved to be of significant value (Kissin and Gross, 1968), current treatment resources are far from adequate (Barton, 1968; Farnsworth, 1968), and family therapy has made a few inroads (Ferreira, 1967). By any of a variety of measures, traditional treatment of alcoholics is not very successful (Pokorny, Miller, and Cleveland, 1968; Tomsovic, 1968).

Traditional psychotherapy, for example, is reported to be effective in less than 18 percent of patients treated for more than one year (Gerard, Saenger, and Wile, 1962). A combination of traditional psychotherapy and physical therapy is the most usual procedure. Assessment of psychotherapeutic efforts tends to fall short of the usual standards of good scientific research (Hill and Blane, 1967) so we may not know the exact efficacy of verbal methods.

Alcoholics Anonymous

Gathering together for mutual support, acceptance, and understanding is one of the aims of Alcoholics Anonymous. The philosophy behind this movement is an outspoken one that rejects personal psychotherapy as an appropriate solution to the problem of remaining sober (Laughlin, 1967). Laughlin suggests that the approach of Alcoholics Anonymous is a repressive and suppressive one that leads to an inspirational, semi-religious rebuilding of life without paying sufficient attention to how the drunk got that way. In rebuttal, the leaders of Alcoholics Anonymous point out that dynamic theory has a poor cure rate.

Dynamic therapists insist the individual must have a penetrating understanding of the how, why, when, and what of the psychological and interpersonal circumstances that produce uncontrolled drinking, i.e., the drunk must understand himself as well as others if he is not to backslide and return to his former state. The credo of Alcoholics Anonymous places emphasis on public confession that the drinker is a "person-with-a-problem," social absolution through confession of one's depraved and deteriorated state, and psychological readiness to accept help from others who have undergone similar experiences.

Approximately one-half of those who come to initial meetings of Alcoholics Anonymous drop out of the organization during the first month. This may be a kind of self-selection that produces among those who remain a close knit group of persons who find the AA method compatible to their nature. Among those who remain and participate regularly, a high rate of recovery is reported. Recovery has only a relative meaning in this context since the AA philosophy suggests that once a drunk, always a drunk and freedom from alcohol must be measured only one day at a time. Recovery from the use of other drugs is measured in much the same way.

Prohibition

Some fifty years ago our society tried a drastic social therapy for alcoholism; it outlawed alcohol in the United States by constitutional amendment. This action failed miserably and in the years between these two alterations of the constitution our country was made the victim of open gang warfare, bootleggers, speak-easies, bathtub gin, and widespread public disregard of the law. Laws became a set of hollow words—words that were unenforceable (Zwerdling and Rosenbaum, 1959).

Despite the lessons painfully learned in the past, a number of states subscribe to peculiar local, restrictive laws with regard to consumption of alcohol in public places, e.g., states in which brown-bagging (bring your own liquor in a brown bag and pay for the glass, ice, and mix the restaurant supplies) is prevalent. States with restrictive legislation about the consumption of food and liquor on the same premises encourage a strange cultural practice, e.g., people gather in private homes to drink for from one to two hours before supper and then careen in a semi-intoxicated condition to a restaurant for the evening meal. These restrictions and their resulting practices are true legal and social anachronisms.

As a society we were forced to face the basic truth about the drug: alcohol, taken in sufficient quantity, relieves anxiety and frees human beings from inhibition. As long as it performs this chemical magic, eliminating it from American social life will be difficult. Some of the young in our society have revolted against the way of life and values of our society by abandoning alcohol and turning to mind distorting drugs such as LSD or the amphetamines. They defend their actions by pointing an accusatory finger at the alcoholic dependence that has long been socially acceptable in our culture (Alexander, 1967; Higgins, 1953).

A few theorists have insisted that the easy access to alcohol in our culture is an obstacle to successful treatment of alcoholics since treatment must contend with a continuous reinforcement for social drinking throughout our society. Since so many drinkers can manage alcohol rather than be managed by it, the root cause must be the interaction of drug and person ready to be drugged. Making alcohol difficult to obtain would simply punish the majority for the symptoms of the minority.

DRUG ADDICTION

Current discussions of drug use in America (Abramson, 1967; Barber, 1967; Klerman, 1968; Louria, 1968; Solomon, 1966) make clear our society's moral and social position with regard to any citizen's right to alter his emotional state or psychological performance by changing his body chemistry. Except for alcohol, tobacco, and caffeine, all important drugs are under medical and legal control and limited to therapeutic uses. The private citizen who smokes marijuana or uses narcotics or LSD does so in defiance of the laws and social ethics of our culture, i.e., no individual has the right to toy with his body's chemical balance. The anti-establishment actions of drug users threaten the prevailing patterns of our society and most often provoke repressive counter-measures from those whose way of life seems in jeopardy.

Drug addiction is usually viewed as symptomatic of personality disorder and is classified as a sociopathic personality disturbance. Categorizing such behavior is far easier than explaining it and recently substantial question has been raised about the sensibleness of trying to differentiate between drug "habituation" and "addiction." One attempt to bring order to the confusion has been that of the Committee on Addiction-Producing Drugs of the World Health Organization. This study committee suggests "drug dependence" might be a more suitable term to encompass the wide range of degrees of addiction. Drug habituation may be an equally appropriate term to describe the phenomenon even though it is unlikely to replace the popular term "addicts."

The opium derivatives, such as morphine or heroin, are the menace our society fears most. The suspected supply route for heroin is an intricate one involving 1. shipping raw opium from Middle Eastern countries to neighboring countries, 2. conversion there into a crude form of morphine, 3. transshipment to yet another country, 4. chemical conversion into heroin, 5. smuggling into the United States, and 6. distribution in a diluted form to the addict. In the first stages of shipment and preparation, the raw material is valued at about $800 a kilogram; sold in small individual packets each kilogram of crude opium may bring as high as $400,000 from addicts. The strength of the final product is so unpredictable, however, that the addict rarely knows the potency of the drug he is using.

Perhaps Wikler (1967) has best blended the present and the future when he said, "Undoubtedly, new drugs of potential dependence will be introduced in the future with a fanfare of statements that they are non-addicting, do not invite drug dependence, and are unassociated with development of tolerance. . . .

"Eventually, the literature will reveal case reports of patients showing intoxication on the drug and an abstinence syndrome at the time of withdrawal. . . .

"It seems equally probable that future antidepressant and stimulating drugs will be abused by some people as a source of 'kicks.' The need for control of drug manufacture and distribution is unlikely ever to end (p. 1010)."

Thus, our present problems forecast those of the immediate and distant future. We must, as a society, decide whether our individual citizens have, within the framework of representative democracy, the right to drug themselves. Until we settle this fundamental philosophic issue, the battle will continue.

When heroin is injected directly into the vein (mainlining), the effect is drowsiness (nodding), euphoria, relief from pain, and a pleasant state seemingly unattainable without the drug (Murray, 1967). Within six hours the effect is gone and the psychological and physiological craving for more returns. If a new supply is unobtainable, withdrawal symptoms begin within 12 hours and, while they vary from addict to addict, at their worst they include vomiting, sneezing, sweating, restlessness, depression, irritability, rapid breathing, alternating hot and cold spells, severe cramps and pains throughout the body, and, at times, hallucinations, or delusions. The physical and emotional peak of withdrawal is passed within three days, most of the symptoms begin to disappear by the fifth day, and the worst sensations are gone by the end of a week. This most extreme form of withdrawal (cold turkey) is not a typical experience for addicts hooked on only moderate daily dosages of the drug. Movie renditions of withdrawal symptoms are dramatized larger than life.

The problem posed by heroin addiction is not that of physical deterioration. Studies of persons addicted for as long as 20 years do not suggest that the drug is physiologically damaging (Pescor, 1944). It is, rather, the addict's obsession with the drug experience and the expense of the habit that contribute significantly to his personal destruction. Some few persons have both affluence and necessary access to drugs to maintain a hidden addiction for extended periods of time. But male addicts steal and women addicts prostitute themselves when money to buy drugs is not available. The life of the deeply addicted derelict human being is regularly recounted in popular periodicals and need not be recounted here. Total dependence on narcotics is a most destructive event in human existence, and our inability to prevent this rush to self-destruction is a mute testimony to the complexity of this happening.

The predominance of Negro drug addiction is a relatively recent phenomenon—in the 1930's most addicts were Caucasians. Today, it is estimated more than one-half of our addicted population is Negro, Mexican, or Puerto Rican; they are young (more than half between 21 and 30 years old); and they are concentrated (nearly 25 percent in the populous states of New York, California, and Illinois). The concentration of addicts clearly is in the large metropolitan areas and equally as clearly is focused in the socially deteriorated inner city. Our drug problem is conjoint with the movement of our poorer citizens into ghetto-like parts of our major cities.

The Dynamics of Addiction

An addict has been described as a person who feels normal only when on drugs. Habituation (a drug-taking habit) suggests a state of psychological dependence on drugs that differs in severity from the obsessive craving and violent physiological reactions experienced when the drug is withdrawn. Habituation can occur for coffee, cigarettes, marijuana, sedatives, tranquilizers, or a variety of stimulants; addiction to any of them is rare.

Theorists seldom suggest addiction is inherited; there is general agreement that the addict learns to use drugs as a means of solving his problems (Gilbert and Lombardi, 1967). Yet, we cannot discover a single, neatly packaged set of personal or social dynamic circumstances invariably associated solely with addiction. We know that "persons-with-problems" discover that the drugged state brings relief from life's difficulties, but this formulation fails to predict who will and will not become an addict. Addiction is a solution to personal psychological difficulties in which it is almost impossible to disentangle cause and effect. Some sociopaths and psychopaths, for example, use drugs in their search for pleasure in much the same fashion that they violate a variety of other social prohibitions. Thus, the addict may have been delinquent before he gets hooked chemically and he continues this delinquent pattern to feed his acquired taste for narcotics (Ausubel, 1961; Clausen, 1957). Or persons restive under the restraints imposed by society may embark on a life of "kicks" and sensual pleasure even if their lives are forfeit in the process.

Addiction is most often portrayed as an illegal, depraved, back-alley way of life. But there are also middle-class addicts who are unable to deal constructively with life's stresses and who seek escape and relief in drugs. The case of Hy R. is illustrative of such a situation.

HY R.

Hy's hands trembled slightly as the needle pricked the vein. He hardly felt it. With his eyes tightly shut, he concentrated on detecting the first signs of the relief he knew morphine would bring. As the surges of relaxation hit him, he shuddered, laughed inwardly, flopped into a chair and visibly began to unwind muscle by muscle. After a few moments he doctored the drug records so that the missing ampule would not be detected. He mused that although Judy was an excellent office nurse, he was just as happy she was pregnant and would be leaving her job in two months. He didn't think she was suspicious yet, but she was smart and you never could be sure. Maybe he would go up north for the deer season and get some rest. Then he could lay off the morphine. Or, at least, cut down on it for awhile.

. . . He had never been a brilliant doctor in anybody's book. But, he figured, most of the people who came to him needed more tender loving care than they did medicine. He worked hard, seldom took a vacation, always answered night calls, and put in longer hours than other doctors. What did they want from him anyway? It seemed as if everyone was on his back. With a sigh he thought again that he never wanted to be a doctor anyway. . . .

He was tired and feeling sorry for himself. He did not know how he got himself into these boxes in life, but he could not remember a time when he was not being pushed by somebody to do things, achieve, accomplish, and get ahead in the world. . . .

Hy had three mental portraits of himself. One image was of himself as others expected him to be. It was a romanticized blending of all that is the best in man. Every virtue was excessive, overstated, and extreme. Hy always hoped that one day he would grow to resemble it more closely than he did at the moment. The second image was a scaled-down, more human version of the first. Its imperfections were apparent, but they were ordinary failings that made it seem more natural. It was the third image that disturbed Hy. It had much more truth in it than the others, but arranged in an ugly and discordant jumble. The total effect was one of imbalance, chaos, and decay. Hy's problem lay in his feeling about this image, which he considered his real self (McNeil, 1967; pp. 137, 138, 139, 140–41).

The sociocultural background of the lower-class addict has greater public visibility. We know the typical addict is liable to be a member of a minority group, the product of a broken home, an inadequate person cut adrift in society with only marginal social connections, and a person suffering from a self-image insufficiently strong to manage his life. We also know he is likely to have been raised in a neighborhood in which poverty, social deterioration, crime, and man's inhumanity to his fellow man prevailed. And we know he has easy access to drugs when other means of coping fail. Most of our information, however, has been acquired from persons *after* they became addicted. We can only surmise and speculate about how it was before drugs made them prisoners. Socially poisonous events spawn a great variety of pathological conditions; drug addiction is only one of them.

Narcotic addiction is the way out most often chosen by members of our lower socioeconomic classes, but other drugs serve the same purpose in the middle class.

LSD

LSD is one of a collection of drugs called the Utopiates by some (Blum, 1964) and the Nightmare Drugs by others (Louria, 1966). LSD-25 (lysergic acid) produces a profound alteration of sensory, perceptual, cognitive, and emotional experiences among its users. And this is the drug of choice among the affluent, educated, middle-class young people in our society (Pearlman, 1967; Pervin, 1967).

The effects of LSD seem to be determined, in part, by the setting in which it is taken and the purposes connected with taking it (Faillace and Szara, 1968). The reaction to LSD in a clinical setting, for example, may be markedly different from that experienced in a clandestine gathering characterized by a cult-like atmosphere of togetherness and illegality (Fort, 1964). The recency of the social upheaval surrounding LSD makes it difficult to recall that this chemical was discovered, by accident, more than a quarter century ago. No one of us then could have predicted the controversy that would surround it or have guessed it would become the preferred drug of the young in our society.

The experience of the LSD user transcends description, but a near approximation may be found in the words of Louria (1966):

> They [colors] swirl around the individual with great vividness. Fixed objects fuse and diffuse; there is often a perpetual flowing of geometric designs and one sensation merges into another and one sense into another so that the individual may say he can taste color; touch sound. The body image is distorted and ordinary sounds increase profoundly in intensity. There is a sense of intense isolation and depersonalization so that "me" as an individual disappears and the user feels he is fused with all humanity and with his environment. Time stands still and many give themselves up to what they describe as an experience of inexpressible ecstasy (pp. 45–46).

It is the opposite of this experience—the "bummer" or "bad trip"—that is so frightening since it produces the kind of total psychological disorganization and disorientation that can only be compared with a full-blown psychosis.

While LSD and heroin are not equally or similarly addictive (there is no evidence LSD is truly addictive), Killam (1964) observes that there are social similarities in its use, i.e., the way users interact with one another, their special language, and their dependency on the drug. The use of LSD allows one to deny the existence of external reality; the user turns inward to private internal emotional experience in the search for truth in life. Consider the case of Bernie F.

BERNIE F.

Bernie was an artsy-craftsy type. She dug origami, esoteric wines, foreign movies, anything high-camp, happenings, total self-expression, and honesty in interpersonal communication. She pitied, but barely tolerated, her other self, candlelighting, husband-hunting, sentiment loving, well-scrubbed, well-mannered, but artificial. Bernie was, with obsessive calculation, all the things her other half was not and she was proud but just a trifle defensive about it. In the first few hours of contact with her I speculated about the possible psychological consequences of her eventual discovery that she unconsciously hungered for the very things she most despised. The tissue separating love and hate is always delicate and easily torn, and it looked as though, in her case, the thin veil was about to be ripped to shreds. . . .

Bernie wants to be a person in her own right and wishes to be treated as a human being first and a woman second. Bernie wants this desperately, but she has serious conflict about accepting either of these roles wholeheartedly. Torn between the middle-class feminine ideal— prim, proper, deodorized, stylized—and its protest version—masculine, unwashed, defiant, long-haired—Bernie was unable to make a clear choice. She viewed society's response to the female as an attempt to cast her in a role subservient to the male. Bernie rebelled against this image of second-class citizenship by denying that she fit the social definition of the female. She looked like a man, she acted like a man, she thought like a man, but she still felt the deep-rooted twinges of femininity within her.

Bernie clearly overreacted to the problems life posed for her and cast her lot with those who, in one form or another, protested but offered no positive, alternative program. For all its mysticism, the fact remains that LSD ingesters are running away from life and hiding from real problems and pressures. Bernie could have involved herself in any number of active social protest movements, but she chose to run from commitment by turning her psychic energies to self-indulgence and introspection. LSD allows its victims to avoid facing problems and this was what Bernie sought most ardently (McNeil, 1967; pp. 117, 121–22).

The use of mind-distorting LSD burst on the American social scene with suddenness that produced immeasurable cultural anxiety and an overreactive upheaval. After a rash of written commentaries, evaluations, and analyses of what was happening (Abramson, 1967; Alpert, Cohen, and Schiller, 1966; Bischoff, 1966; Cashman, 1966; Goldstein, 1966; Leary, Metzner, and Alpert, 1964; Masters and Houston, 1966; Solomon, 1964) LSD was treated as addicting in the usual sense of traditional opiates. Yet, dependence on the drug was not clearly established and, even today,

it is not the relaxant of choice of the older generation. On moral grounds it might be argued that human kind already has more than a sufficiency of drugs available to quell its anxieties and relieve its tensions. But, the morality of chemical alteration of consciousness is hard-pressed and cannot sensibly be stretched to encompass the legal sanction of one chemical coupled with a remarkable legal oppression of another. It is evident that the issue of the chemistry of happiness will concern our society for some years to come.

For some few, marijuana will be the precursor to a life of addiction to hard narcotics; for most, it will be an end in itself and will not lead to self-destruction. Our ability to predict which fate is in store for the individual marijuana smoker is, however, grossly imperfect at this stage.

Sedatives, Tranquilizers, and Stimulants

The chemical industries of this country manufacture more than 13 billion tranquilizers, sedatives, and stimulants to be dispensed by more than 50,000 drug stores. We are well-described as a nation of pill-taking hypochondriacs bombarded by urgings to drugged escape from the troubles of a complex technological society (Louria, 1966). The numbers of our citizens dependent on drugs amount to 20 million, and the legitimate and illegitimate profits gleaned from the drug traffic are counted in the hundreds of millions of dollars. New drugs appear on the market each week and chemical magic has become a common and convenient way to satisfy troubled patients.

While it is handy to describe sedatives, tranquilizers, and stimulants as though each had a single effect, this seldom is the case. The first therapeutic stimulants, for example, made patients more "reactive" to stimuli around them yet did little to change the content of their thoughts and perceptions. There is no drug that acts on behavior alone. All drugs alter the individual's internal physical balance and the action of the drug differs from its effect. Thus, tranquilizers (ataractics) are designed to quell anxiety but there may be a sedative side effect in their action. The individual may not be able to distinguish between being tranquil or merely sleepy.

Sedatives are derivatives of barbiturate acids which produce relaxation and reduction of tension. Taken in moderation these drugs appear harmless. Taken in excess they produce intellectual and muscular deterioration. As habituation occurs, the dosage level must be increased until the amount is so great that the drug-taker endangers his life. The combination of alcohol and barbiturates is reported to be particularly lethal.

Sedatives were first used medically as a form of chemical restraint to replace physical restraints, i.e., strait-jackets long in use in asylums (Sharoff, 1967). The use of these sedatives was soon extended to the treatment of patients of all kinds by continuous sedation for extended periods of time. Today sedatives such as Nembutal, Amytal, and Pheno-barbital are widely used to take the sting out of rage, anxiety, guilt, and unhappiness. Sedatives are freely used by some physicians to help patients meet each and every crisis situation in which emotional stress is being experienced.

In the decade and a half since the discovery and refinement of tran-quilizers there has been a spectacular increase in the rate of their pre-scription and ingestion (Ewing, 1967). We take major and minor tran-quilizers at a rate of millions of pounds each year and the upper limit has yet to be reached. Yet, habituation to tranquilizers is rarer than to the barbiturates.

The tranquilizers are usually subdivided into major and minor or strong and weak categories. The major tranquilizers consist of the *Phenothiazines* (commercially named Sparine, Mellaril, Stelazine, Thorazine, or Compa-zine, etc.) and the *Rauwolfia Alkaloids* (commercially named Sepasil, Harmonyl, Moderil, Raudixin, etc.). The minor tranquilizers have a great many names; the most familiar of which may be Librium, Miltown, or Equanil. Such tranquilizers are thought to make up about 10 percent of the nearly 65 million prescriptions dispensed each year by pharmacists. For the general practitioner of medicine, tranquilizing agents make up the third most common drug prescribed. The bulk of tranquility pills administered to calm our society is made up of minor tranquilizers. Sur-prisingly, there is no reliable evidence that these minor tranquilizers are any better than the harmless sugar-coated placebos.

The tranquilizers are probably improperly named (Denber, 1967). They do make agitated patients more "tranquil" but, as we noted in Chapter Four, it is the progressive disappearance of symptoms in acute and chronic emotional disorders that makes the "tranquilizers" so valuable. Tranquilizers are used with almost all kinds of disorder. Denber's list of symptoms so treatable (regardless of diagnosis) includes tension, anxiety, hyperactivity, agitation, impulsiveness, aggressiveness, and audi-tory or visual hallucinations.

In the late 1950's the stimulants or antidepressant drugs were dis-covered as an accidental byproduct of the search for improved tran-quilizers. These new stimulants, or euphoria-producers, had no significant effect when administered to "normals" but they acted to lift deep depres-sion and allowed the medical profession to take an important therapeutic stride forward. Mood-elevators in use previously often had severe side-reactions (jumpiness, insomnia, or loss of appetite) and the induced euphoria lasted only a few hours before an even deeper depression occurred.

Stimulants (the amphetamines, benzedrine, dexedrine, dexamyl, methedrine) may, if taken in sufficient quantity for a long enough time, produce serious consequences. The initial feeling of exhilaration and euphoria may culminate in confused, irrational, paranoid, hallucinatory, and delusional thoughts. Stimulants do not addict, as do the opiates, and withdrawal symptoms may not be experienced by the user unless the dose has been heavy and the withdrawal abrupt. The tranquilizers, sedatives, and stimulants do produce a vicious cycle of agitation and relief and it is this cycle that is so difficult to break. In various combinations, these drugs can alter the body chemistry and keep the user constantly detached from normal existence.

The Treatment of Drug Addiction

Treatment of drug addiction is a particularly difficult challenge, a challenge that has been met with little success (Levitt, 1968). Prevention is always the preferred course of action, but we know too little of the exact dynamics of addiction and we are frequently confronted with social pressures that demand punishment for this transgression rather than treatment of it.

Flat withdrawal from the drugged state has proved to be effective only for a short period of time for most addicts. Detoxification, whether done suddenly or over an extended period of time, will never be the sole answer if 90 percent of the patients become readdicted shortly after release from the hospital (Hunt and Odoroff, 1962; Duvall, Locke, and Brill, 1963). Substitution of a less addictive drug (Methadone), for example, is "maintenance therapy" but the reasoning at the base of this method has been called self-defeating and circular since it does not address itself to the causes of addiction. Rather, it substitutes one drug for another.

Hopefully, a nonaddicting substitute for heroin will one day be discovered. Theorists have pointed out that this is probably a gross contradiction in terms since the search for pleasure, escape, and relief is what drives the potential addict to drugs and if new, nonaddictive drugs fail to provide these pleasures they cannot become a substitute. It is unlikely we will find a joy-filled chemical compound that is neither physiologically or psychologically addictive.

Aversive therapy has also been attempted. Apomorphine has been mixed with morphine to produce nausea in contact with the drug, for example. But the results reported even for limited addict samples have been less than promising (Liberman, 1968). As with the alcoholics, a powerful need for the drug will overcome even nausea.

Similar to Alcoholics Anonymous, a movement called Synanon (a word coined by an addict who could not pronounce "symposium") was formed in 1958 in California to assist the addict population. This movement establishes therapeutic communities of addicts who live on a communal basis (Yablonsky, 1963, 1967). To succeed in this new way of life (as many as 50 percent of the addicts fail to make it), the individual must be well motivated to abandon his old life and able to accept a rigid and authoritarian (almost cult-like) new pattern of living. Each addict helps other users stay clean of drugs as he becomes a therapist teaching new members to relate to the system and communicate their feelings.

Synanon is an interpersonal, group-oriented means of establishing a "clean" subculture with a set of values and standards of behavior that can counteract those of the neighborhood in which the addiction was first formed. Typically, drugs offer the young person a way of avoiding rather than solving problems; drug use is a way of rejecting the demands and values of society while postponing a final decision about them until another day (Levy, 1968).

Addiction may begin as an expression of a "hang-loose" ethic that rejects establishment values (Suchman, 1968). This ethic may be incorporated into the life-style of the child in such a way that he experiments with drugs in order to establish his image as a "stand-up cat" who is not afraid of anything. The group support he receives for such daring enterprise may only be diminished if he can become a part of a social group that rejects self-drugging as an answer to life's problems—a group such as Synanon. The Synanon group offers him a way to avoid the relapse that is so often the fate of his fellow addict (Akers, Burgess, Johnson, 1968).

Still, broad social attitudes must be changed with regard to addiction before much progress can be achieved (Bowman, 1958). Until the forces that drive the individual to drugs are remedied and until he is viewed sympathetically as a person-with-a-problem, little progress will be made. The present punitive official approach drives the addict into hiding and to a life of crime and dissolution to support his habit.

Trends in public attitudes to narcotic addiction have not remained static; they have changed with the times (Pattison, Bishop, and Linsky, 1968). Articles in popular magazines over the past seven decades, reveal that the addict is now viewed as less responsible for his behavior, more a victim of his social surroundings, and there has been some softening in public punitive attitudes and a turn to emphasis on medical and social rehabilitation.

SUMMARY

The disruption to orderly social life produced by personality disorders and trait disturbances is probably most clearly exemplified by those in our society who become addicted to pharmocological or chemical forms of escape from the problems of living. Alcohol has proven to be the most problematical of drugs since its use is widespread, sanctioned, and reinforced by the culture despite the fact that its excessive use exacts an exceptional psychological, social, and economic toll.

Persons become problem drinkers as a learned dynamic response to interpersonal and social pressures that force them to use defensive psychological distortions of real life. Their inability to manage tension in a mature fashion is marked by both a deep dependency and fundamental hostility directed toward those close to them.

Addiction to hard narcotic drugs is dynamically related to the choice of alcohol as a means of escape from life's tensions, but it differs by being a phenomenon most apparent in the lowest socioeconomic level in our society. Drugs most often serve as a way out for oppressed and mistreated members of minority groups. Hard narcotic addiction is so clearly self-destructive that it must be viewed as an act of psychic desperation on the part of a small number of inadequate personalities for whom the harsh realities of living simply prove overwhelming.

Habituation to the nonaddictive drugs (LSD, sedatives, tranquilizers, and stimulants) is widespread in our anxiety-laden culture and poses an equally great but less visible problem. Such drugs alter but do not seriously distort the human chemical balance and, thus, are reacted to with less social alarm.

Therapeutic efforts have not produced much to offer hope for remedy of this form of social deviation. The motivation behind serious addiction seems learned early enough to be so deeply entrenched that it seriously limits efforts to eliminate or eradicate it. Addiction may prove to be the least tractable of all the personality disorders and trait disturbances.

References

ABRAMSON, H. (ed.), *The Use of LSD in Psychotherapy and Alcoholism.* Indianapolis, Ind.: The Bobbs-Merrill Co., Inc., 1967.

ABT, L. E., and S. L. WEISSMAN, *Acting Out.* New York: Grune & Stratton, Inc., 1965.

AKERS, R. L., R. L. BURGESS, and W. T. JOHNSON, Opiate use, addiction and relapse. *Social Problems,* 1968, *15,* 459–69.

ALBERT, R. S., T. R. BRIGANTE, and M. CHASE, The psychopathic personality: a content analysis of the concept. *J. gen. Psych.,* 1950, *60,* 17–28.

ALEXANDER, F., *Psychosomatic Medicine: Its Principles and Application.* New York: W. W. Norton & Co., Inc., 1950.

ALEXANDER, F. G., and S. T. SELESNICK, *The History of Psychiatry.* New York, N.Y.: Harper & Row, Publishers, 1965.

ALEXANDER, C. N., Alcohol and adolescent rebellion. *Soc. Forces,* 1967, *45,* 542–50.

ALLEN, C., *A Textbook of Psychosexual Disorders.* London: Oxford University Press, 1962.

ALLPORT, G. W., *Personality, A Psychological Interpretation.* New York: Holt, Rinehart & Winston, Inc., 1937.

ALPERT, R., S. COHEN, and L. SCHILLER, *LSD.* New York: New American Library, 1966.

ANDREWS, J. W., Psychotherapy of phobias. *Psych. Bull.,* 1966, *66,* 455–80.

ANTHONY, E. J., Psychoneurotic disorders. In *Psychiatry,* A. M. Freedman and H. I. Kaplan (eds.). Baltimore, Md.: Williams and Wilkins, 1967, pp. 1387–1406.

APPERSON, LOUISE B., and W. G. McADOO, Parental factors in the childhood of homosexuals. *J. Abnorm. Psychol.,* 1968, *73,* 201–6.

ARGYRIS, C., T-groups for organizational effectiveness. *Harvard Business Review*, 1964, *42*, 60–74.

ARIETI, S., *The Intrapsychic Self*. New York: Basic Books, Inc., Publishers, 1967.

AUSUBEL, D. P., Causes and types of narcotic addiction: a psychosocial view. *Psychiat. Quart.*, 1961, *35*, 523–31.

AVERILL, J. R., Grief: its nature and significance. *Psych. Bull.*, 1968, *70*, 721–48.

BALES, R. F., Cultural differences in rates of alcoholism. *Quart. J. Stud. Alcohol*, 1946, *6*, 480–99.

BANDURA, A., and R. H. WALTERS, *Adolescent Aggression*. New York: The Ronald Press Company, 1959.

BARBER, B., *Drugs and Society*. New York: Russell Sage Foundation, 1967.

BARTON, W. E., Deficits in the treatment of alcoholism and recommendations for correction. *Amer. J. Psychiatr.*, 1968, *124*, 1679–86.

BECK, A. T., *Depression*. New York: Harper & Row, Publishers, 1967.

BEHRING, D. W., and S. L. BRUNING, Concept formation and the psychopathic personality. *J. Special Educ.*, 1967, *2*, 105–10.

BENDA, C. E., Neurosis of conscience. *J. Existentialism*, 1967, *7*, 425–42.

BERECZ, J. M., Phobias of childhood: Etiology and treatment. *Psychol. Bull.*, 1968, *70*, 694–720.

BERG, I. A., Observations concerning obsessive tunes in normal persons under stress. *J. clin. Psychol.*, 1953, 9, 300–302.

BERGLER, E., *Homosexuality, Disease or Way of Life*. New York: Hill and Wang, 1956.

BERNARD, J. L., and R. EISENMAN, Verbal conditioning in sociopaths with social and monetary reinforcement. *J. pers. soc. Psychol.*, 1967, *6*, 203–6.

BIEBER, I., *Homosexuality*. New York: Basic Books, Inc., Publishers, 1962.

BIEBER, I., Sexual deviations: Introduction. In *Psychiatry*, A. M. Freedman and H. I. Kaplan (eds.). Baltimore, Md.: Williams and Wilkins, 1967, pp. 959–62.

BISCHOFF, W. H., *The Ecstasy Drugs*. Delray Beach, Fla.: Circle Press, 1966.

BLAKEMORE, C. B., J. G. THORPE, J. C. BARKER, C. G. CONWAY, and N. I. LAVIN, The application of faradic aversion conditioning in a case of transvestism. *Behaviour Research and Therapy*, 1963, *1*, 29–34.

BLANE, L., and R. H. ROTH, Voyeurism and exhibitionism. *Percept. Mot. Skills*, 1967, *24*, 391–400.

BLOCK, JEANNE, ELINOR HARVEY, P. H. JENNINGS, and ELAINE SIMPSON, Clinicians' conceptions of the asthmatogenic mother. *Arch. gen. Psychiatr.*, 1966, *15*, 610–18.

BLUM, R., *et al.*, *Utopiates*. New York, N. Y.: Atherton Press, 1964.

BONIME, W., The Psychodynamics of neurotic depression. In *American Handbook of Psychiatry*, S. Arieti (ed.). New York: Basis Books, Inc., Publisher, 1966, pp. 239–55.

BOWMAN, K. M., Some problems of addiction. In *Psychopathology of Communication*, P. Hoch and J. Zubin (eds.). New York: Grune & Stratton, Inc., 1958.

BRANCALE, R., A. ELLIS, and RUTH DOORBAR, Psychiatric and psychological investigations of convicted sex offenders: a summary report. *Amer. J. Psychiatr.*, 1952, *109*, 17–21.

BREGER, L., and J. L. McGAUGH, Critique and reformulation of "learning theory" approaches to psychotherapy and neurosis. *Psych. Bull.*, 1965, *63*, 338–58.

BRODY, E. B., and L. S. SATA, Trait and pattern disturbances. In *Psychiatry*, A. M. Freedman and H. I. Kaplan (eds.). Baltimore, Md.: Williams and Wilkins, 1967, 937–50.

BROSIN, H. W., Brain syndromes associated with trauma. In *Psychiatry*, A. M. Freedman and H. I. Kaplan (eds.). Baltimore, Md.: Williams and Wilkins, 1967, pp. 748–59.

BUSS, A. H., *Psychopathology*. New York: John Wiley & Sons, Inc., 1966.

BUSSE, E. W., Brain syndromes associated with disturbances in metabolism, growth and nutrition. In *Psychiatry*, A. M. Freedman and H. I. Kaplan (eds.). Baltimore, Md.: Williams and Wilkins, 1967, 726–39.

CABEEN, C. W., and J. C. COLEMAN, Group therapy with sex offenders: description and evaluation of group therapy program. *J. Clin. Psychol.*, 1961, *17*, 122–29.

CAMERON, N., *Personality Development and Psychopathology*. Boston: Houghton Mifflin Company, 1963.

CAMPBELL, J. P., and M. D. DUNNETTE, Effectiveness of T-Group experiences in managerial training and development. *Psych. Bull.*, 1968, *70*, 73–104.

CAREY, J. T., and J. MANDEL, A San Francisco Bay Area "speed" scene. *J. Health and Social Behavior*, 1968, *9*, 164–74.

CASHMAN, J., *The LSD Story*. Greenwich, Conn.: Fawcett, 1966.

CAVAN, SHERRI, *Liquor License*. Chicago: Aldine Publishing Co., 1966.

CHAFETZ, M. E., Addictions. III: Alcoholism. In *Psychiatry*, A. M. Freedman and H. I. Kaplan (eds.). Baltimore, Md.: Williams and Wilkins, 1967, pp. 1011–26.

CHRISTOFFEL, H., Male genital exhibitionism. In *Perversions: Psychodynamics and Therapy*, S. Lorand, and M. Bolint (eds.). New York: Random House, Inc., 1956, pp. 243–64.

CHURCHILL, W., *Homosexual Behavior Among Males: A Cross-Cultural and Cross-Species Investigation*. New York: Hawthorn Books, Inc., 1967.

CLAUSEN, J. A., Social patterns, personality and adolescent drug use. In *Explorations in Social Psychiatry*, A. H. Leighton, J. A. Clausen, and R. N. Wilson (eds.). New York: Basic Books, Inc., Publishers, 1957.

CLECKLEY, H., *The Mask of Sanity*. St. Louis: Mosby, 1955.

CLECKLEY, H. M., Psychopathic states. In *American Handbook of Psychiatry*, S. Arieti (ed.). New York: Basic Books, Inc., Publishers, 1959, 567–88.

COLE, J. O., and J. M. DAVIS, Antidepressant drugs. In *Psychiatry*, A. M. Freedman and H. I. Kaplan (eds.). Baltimore, Md.: Williams and Wilkins, 1967, pp. 1203–75.

COLEMAN, J. C., *Abnormal Psychology and Modern Life* (3rd ed.). Chicago: Scott, Foresman & Company, 1964.

CONGER, J. J., The effects of alcohol on conflict behavior in the albino rat. *Quart. J. Stud. Alcohol,* 1951, *12,* 1–29.

CONGER, J. J., Reinforcement theory and the dynamics of alcoholism. *Quart. J. Stud. Alcohol,* 1956, *17,* 296–305.

COPPOLINO, C. A., and CARMELA M. COPPOLINO, *The Billion Dollar Hangover.* New York: Popular Library, 1965.

CURLEE, JOAN, Alcoholic women: some considerations for further research. *Bull. Menninger Clin.,* 1967, *31,* 154–63.

CUTNER, MARGOT, The use of LSD 25 in psychotherapy and some ideas on its function in drug-addiction. *Psychotherapy and Psychosomatics,* 1967, *15,* 14.

DARLING, H. F., Definition of psychopathic personality. *J. nerv. Ment. Dis.,* 1945, *10,* 121–26.

DARLING, H. F., and J. W. SANDDAL, A psychopathologic concept of psychopathic personality. *J. Clin. Exper. Psychopathol.,* 1952, *13,* 175–80.

DAVIDS, A., M. JOELSON, and C. McARTHUR, Rorschach and TAT indices of homosexuality in overt homosexuals, neurotics and normal males. *J. abnorm. soc. Psychol.,* 1956, *53,* 161–72.

DAVIS, F., and LAURA NUMOZ, Heads and freaks: Patterns and meanings of drug use among hippies. *J. Health & Social Behavior,* 1968, *9,* 156–64.

DAVIS, F. B., The relationship between suicide and attempted suicide: a review of the literature. *Psychiatric Quart.,* 1967, *41,* 752–65.

DAVIS, F. B., Sex differences in suicide and attempted suicide. *Dis. Nerv. Syst.,* 1968, *29,* 193–94.

DENBER, H. C. B., Tranquilizers in psychiatry. In *Psychiatry,* A. M. Freedman and H. I. Kaplan (eds.). Baltimore, Md.: Williams and Wilkins, 1967, pp. 1251–63.

DENT, J. Y., Dealing with the alcoholic at home. *Med. World Lond.,* 1954, *81,* 245.

DERI, S. K., A problem in obesity. *Clinical Studies of Personality.* New York: Harper and Row, Publishers, 1955.

DEVEREAUX, G., Cultural factors in therapy. *J. of Amer. Psychoanal. Assoc.,* 1953, *1,* 643–55.

Diagnostic and Statistical Manual, Mental Disorders, American Psychiatric Assoc., Mental Hospital Service, Washington, D.C., 1952.

DIXON, J. J., CECILY DEMONCHAUX, and J. SANDLER, Patterns of anxiety: the phobias. *British J. of Medical Psychology,* 1957, *30,* 34–40.

DOIDGE, W. T., and W. H. HOLTZMAN, Implications of homosexuality among Air Force trainees. *J. consult. Psychol.,* 1960, *24,* 9–14.

DUNBAR, H. F., *Emotions and Bodily Changes.* New York: Columbia University Press, 1946.

DUNHAM, H. W., *Crucial Issues in the Treatment and Control of Sexual Deviation in the Community.* Lansing, Mich.: State Department of Mental Health, 1951.

DUVALL, H. J., B. Z. LOCKE, and L. BRILL, Follow-up study of narcotics drug addicts five years after hospitalization. *Publ. Hlth. Rep.,* 1963, *78,* 185–93.

EAST, W. N., Sexual offenders. *J. nerv. ment. Dis.*, 1946, *103*, 626–66.

ELLIS, A., and A. ABARNEL (EDS.), *The Encyclopedia of Sexual Behavior* (Vols. I & II). New York: Hawthorn Books, Inc., 1961.

ELLIS, H., *Studies in the Psychology of Sex*. New York: Random House, Inc., 1942.

ENGLISH, O. S., Education in mental health combined with treatment of psychosomatic illness. *Psychotherapy and Psychosomatics*, 1967, *15*, 135–41.

EVANS, D. R., Masturbatory fantasy and sexual deviation. *Behaviour Research and Therapy*, 1968, *6*, 17–19.

EWING, J. A., Addiction. II: Non-narcotic addictive agents. In *Psychiatry*, A. M. Freedman and H. I. Kaplan (eds.). Baltimore, Md.: Williams and Wilkins, 1967, pp. 1003–11.

EYSENCK, H. J., *Behaviour Therapy and the Neuroses*. London: Pergamon Press, 1960.

FAILLACE, L. A., and S. SZARA, Hallucinogenic drugs: Influence of mental set and setting. *Disease of the Nervous System*, 1968, *29*, 124–26.

FARBEROW, N. L., and E. S. SCHNEIDMAN, *The Cry for Help*. New York: McGraw-Hill Book Company, 1961.

FARNSWORTH, D. L., Medical perspectives on alcoholism and around-the-clock psychiatric services. *Amer. J. Psychiatr.*, 1968, *124*, 1659–63.

FELDMAN, H. W., Ideological supports to becoming and remaining a heroin addict. *J. of Health & Social Behavior*, 1968, *9*, 131–39.

FELDMAN, M. P., Aversion therapy for sexual deviations: A critical review. *Psych. Bull.*, 1966, *65*, 65–79.

FENICHEL, O., *The Psychoanalytic Theory of Neurosis*. New York: W. W. Norton & Company, Inc., 1945.

FERREIRA, A. J., Family therapy in alcoholism. *Psychotherapy and Psychosomatics*, 1967, *15*, 20.

FITZELLE, G. T., Personality factors and certain attitudes toward child rearing among parents of asthmatic children. *Psychosom. Med.*, 1959, *21*, 208–17.

FORD, C. S., and F. A. BEACH, *Patterns of Sexual Behavior*. New York: Harper & Row, Publishers, 1951.

FORD, R. M., The treatment of intractable childhood asthma by medium-term separation from home environment. *Medical J. of Australia*, 1968, *1*, 653–56.

FOREST, T., Paternal roots of male character development. *Psychoanalyt. Rev.*, 1967, *54*, 51–68.

FORT, J., Social and legal response to pleasure giving drugs. In *Utopiates*, R. Blum, *et al.* (eds.). New York: Atherton Press, 1964, pp. 205–23.

FRANK, J. D., The dynamics of the psychotherapeutic relationship: Determinants and effects of the therapist's influence. *Psychiatry*, 1959, *22*, 17–39.

FRANK, J. D. *Persuasion and healing: A comparative study of psychotherapy*. Baltimore: Johns Hopkins Press, 1961.

FRANKENSTEIN, C., *Psychopathy—A Comparative Analysis of Clinical Pictures*. New York: Grune & Stratton, Inc., 1959.

FRAZIER, S. H., and A. C. CARR, Phobic reaction. In *Psychiatry*, A. M. Freedman and H. I. Kaplan (eds.). Baltimore, Md.: Williams and Wilkins, 1967, pp. 899–911.

FREEDMAN, A. M., and ETHEL A. WILSON, Sociopathic personality disorders. III: Addiction and alcoholism. In *Psychiatry*, A. M. Freedman and H. I. Kaplan (eds.). Baltimore, Md.: Williams and Wilkins, 1967, pp. 1429–32.

FREEDMAN, MARCIA K., Sociopathic personality disorders. I: Sociological aspects of juvenile delinquency. In *Psychiatry*, A. M. Freedman and H. I. Kaplan (eds.). Baltimore, Md.: Williams and Wilkins, 1967, pp. 1424–26.

FREEMAN, E. H., B. F. FEINGOLD, K. SCHLESINGER, and F. J. GORMAN, Psychological variables in allergic disorders: A review. *Psychosom. Med.*, 1964, *26*, 543–75.

FREUD, S., Three contributions to the theory of sex. In *The Collected Writings of Sigmund Freud*, A. A. Brill (ed.). New York: Modern Library, Inc., 1938.

FREUD, S., The psychogenesis of a case of homosexuality in a woman. *Collected Papers*, Vol. 2. New York: Basic Books, Inc., Publishers, 1959, pp. 202–31.

FRIBERG, R. R., Measures of homosexuality: cross-validation of two MMPI scales and implications for usage. *J. consult. Psychol.*, 1967, *31*, 88–91.

FRIEDMAN, A. P., Headache. In *Psychiatry*, A. M. Freedman and H. I. Kaplan (eds.). Baltimore, Md.: Williams and Wilkins Co., 1967, pp. 1110–13.

FRIEDMAN, M., James Baldwin and psychotherapy. *Psychotherapy: Theory, Research and Practice*, 1966, *3*, 177–83.

FRIEDMAN, P., Sexual deviations. In *American Handbook of Psychiatry*, S. Arieti (ed.). New York: Basic Books, Inc., Publishers, 1959, pp. 589–613.

FROMM, E., *Man for Himself*. New York: Rinehart, 1947.

GELDER, M. G., and I. M. MARKS, Desensitization and phobias: A crossover study. *Brit. J. Psychiat.*, 1968, *114*, 323–28.

GERARD, D. L., G. SAENGER, and R. WILE, The Abstinent Alcoholic. *Arch. Gen. Psychiat.*, 1962, *6*, 83–95.

GIBBONS, D. C., *Changing the Lawbreaker*. Englewood Cliffs, N.J.: Prentice-Hall, Inc., 1965.

GILBERT, JEANNE G., and D. N. LOMBARDI, Personality characteristics of young male narcotic addicts. *J. consult. Psychol.*, 1967, *31*, 536–38.

GINSBURG, K. N., The "meat-rack": A study of the male homosexual prostitute. *Amer. J. Psychother.*, 1967, *21*, 170–85.

GLUECK, S., and E. GLUECK, *Unraveling Juvenile Delinquency*. Cambridge, Mass.: Harvard Univer. Press, 1950.

GLUECK, B. C., JR., *Final Report, Research Project for the Study and Treatment of Persons Convicted of Crime Involving Sexual Aberrations*. New York: State Dept. of Ment. Hyg., 1956.

GODFREY, L., M. D. KISSEN, and T. M. DOWNS, Treatment of the acute alcohol-withdrawal syndrome. *Quart. J. Stud. Alcohol*, 1958, *19*, 118–24.

GOLDSTEIN, R., *1 in 7: Drugs on Campus*. New York: Walker and Co., 1966.

GOMBERG, EDITH S. L., Etiology of alcoholism. *J. consult. & clin. Psychol.*, 1968, *32*, 18–20.

GRANT, V. W., A case study of fetishism. *J. abnorm. soc. Psychol.*, 1953, *48*, 142–49.

GREEN, E., D. SILVERMAN, and G. GEIL, Petit mal electro-shock therapy of criminal psychopaths. *J. Crim. Psychopathol.*, 1943, *5*, 667–73.

GREENACRE, PHYLLIS, Conscience in the psychopath. *Amer. J. Orthopsychiat.*, 1945, *15*, 495–509.

GREENWALD, H., Treatment of the psychopath. *Voices*, 1967, *3*, 50–60.

GREGORY, J., *Fundamentals of Psychiatry*. Philadelphia: W. B. Saunders Co., 1968.

GUTTMACHER, M. S., *Sex Offenses: The Problem, Cause and Prevention*. New York: W. W. Norton & Company, Inc., 1961.

HAHN, W. W., and JEAN A. CLARK, Psychophysiological reactivity of asthmatic children. *Psychosomatic Med.*, 1967, *29*, 526–36.

HALD, J., and E. JACOBSEN, A drug sensitizing the organism to ethyl alcohol. *Lancet*, 1948, ii, 1001.

HALLECK, S. L., Emotional effects of victimization. In *Sexual Behavior and the Law*, R. Slovenko (ed.). Springfield, Ill.: Charles C Thomas, Publishers, 1965, pp. 673–86.

HALLECK, S. L., *Psychiatry and the Dilemmas of Crime*. New York: Hoeber Medical Books, 1967.

HARE, R. D., Psychopathy, fear arousal and anticipated pain. *Psych. Rep.*, 1965, *16*, 499–502.

HARTUNG, F., *Crime, Law and Society*. Detroit: Wayne University Press, 1965.

HAVIGHURST, R. J., and HILDA TABA, *Adolescent Character and Personality*. New York: John Wiley & Sons, Inc., 1949.

HEATON-WARD, W. A., Psychopathic disorder. *Lancet*, 1963, *1*, 121–23.

HEIDENSOHN, FRANCES, The deviance of women: a critique and an enquiry. *Brit. J. Sociol.*, 1968, *19*, 160–75.

HEINE, R. W. (ed.), *The Student Physician as Psychotherapist*. Chicago: The University of Chicago Press, 1962.

HENDIN, H., Suicide. In *Psychiatry*, A. M. Freedman and H. I. Kaplan (eds.). Baltimore, Md.: Williams and Wilkins Co., 1967, pp. 1170–79.

HENDRICK, I., *Facts and Theories of Psychoanalysis* (3rd ed.). New York: Alfred A. Knopf, Inc., 1958.

HENNINGER, J. M., Exhibitionism. *J. crim. Psychopath.*, 1941, *2*, 357–66.

HERBERT, M., R. GLICK, and H. BLACK, Olfactory precipitants of bronchial asthma. *J. Psychosomatic Res.*, 1967, *11*, 195–202.

HERSKOVITZ, H. H., M. LEVINE, and G. SPIVAK, Anti-social behavior of adolescents from higher socio-economic groups. *J. Nerv. & Ment. Dis.*, 1959, *129*, 467–76.

HETHERINGTON, E. MAVIS, and E. KLINGER, Psychopathy and punishment. *J. abnorm. soc. Psychol.*, 1964, *69*, 113–15.

HIGGINS, J. W., Psychodynamics in the excessive drinking of alcohol. *Arch. Neurol. Psychiat.*, 1953, *69*, 713–17.

HILL, MARJORIE J., and H. T. BLANE, Evaluation of psychotherapy with alcoholics. *Quart. J. Stud. Alcohol*, 1967, *28*, 76–104.

HOLLAND, B. C., and R. S. WARD, Homeostasis and psychosomatic medicine. In *American Handbook of Psychiatry*, S. Arieti (ed.). New York: Basic Books, Inc., 1966, pp. 344–61.

HOLLIDAY, A. R., A review of psychopharmacology. In *Handbook of Clinical Psychology*, B. B. Wolman (ed.). New York: McGraw-Hill Book Co., 1965, pp. 1296–1322.

HOOKER, EVELYN, The adjustment of the male overt homosexual. *J. proj. Tech.*, 1957, *21*, 18–31.

HOOKER, EVELYN, Male homosexuality in the Rorschach. *J. proj. Tech.*, 1958, *22*, 35–54.

HOOKER, EVELYN, Male homosexuality. In *Taboo Topics*, N. L. Farberow (ed.). New York: Atherton Press, 1963, pp. 44–55.

HOPPE, K. D., J. MOLNAR, J. NEWELL, and A. LAND, Diagnostic and developmental classifications of adolescent offenders. *Comprehensive Psychiatr.*, 1967, *8*, 277–83.

HORNEY, KAREN, *Our Inner Conflicts*. New York: W. W. Norton & Company, Inc., 1945.

HORTON, D., The functions of alcohol in primitive societies: a cross-cultural study. *Quart. J. Stud. Alcohol*, 1943, *4*, 199–220.

HUNT, G. H., and M. E. ODOROFF, Follow-up study of narcotic addicts after hospitalization. *Publ. Hlth. Rep.*, 1962, *77*, 41–54.

HUNTER, H., Kleinfeter's syndrome and delinquency. *British J. of Criminology*, 1968, *8*, 203–7.

ISBELL, H., Craving for alcohol. *Quart. J. Stud. Alcohol*, 1955, *16*, 38–42.

JACOBS, M. A., *et al.*, Incidence of psychosomatic predisposing factors in allergic disorders. *Psychosomatic Med.*, 1966, *28*, 679–95.

JANIS, I. L., G. F. MAHL, J. KAGAN, and R. R. HOLT, *Personality*. New York: Harcourt, Brace & World, Inc., 1969.

JELLINEK, E. M., Phases of alcohol addiction. *Quart. J. Stud. Alcohol*, 1952, *13*, 673–78.

JELLINEK, E. M., *The Disease Concept of Alcoholism*. New Haven, Conn.: Hillhouse Press, 1960.

JONES, M., *The Therapeutic Community—A New Treatment Method in Psychiatry*. New York: Basic Books, Inc., Publishers, 1953.

JONES, MARY C., The elimination of children's fears. *J. Exp. Psych.*, 1924, *7*, 382–90.

JONES, MARY C., Personality correlates and antecedents of drinking patterns in adult males. *J. consult. & clin. Psychol.*, 1968, *32*, 2–12.

JOSSELYN, IRENE, Acting out in adolescence. In *Acting Out*, L. E. Abt and S. L. Weissman (eds.). New York: Grune & Stratton, Inc., 1965, pp. 68–75.

KAHN, M., and B. BAKER, Desensitization with minimal therapist contact. *J. abnorm. Psychol.*, 1968, *73*, 198–200.

KALIS, BETTY L., R. E. HARRIS, M. SOKOLOW, and L. G. CARPENTER, Response to psychological stress in patients with essential hypertension. *Amer. Heart J.*, 1957, *53*, 572–78.

KAPLAN, H. I., History of psychosomatic medicine. In *Psychiatry*, A. M. Freedman and H. I. Kaplan (eds.). Baltimore, Md.: Williams and Wilkins Co., 1967, pp. 1036–37.

KARDINER, A., *The Individual and His Society*. New York: Columbia Univer. Press, 1939.

KARPMAN, B., On the need for separating psychopathy into two distinct clinical types: Symptomatic and idiopathic. *J. crim. & Psychopath.*, 1941, *3*, 112–37.

KARPMAN, B., *The Sexual Offender and His Offenses*. New York: Julian Press, 1954.

KAYTON, L., and G. F. BORGE, Birth order and the obsessive-compulsive character. *Arch. Gen. Psychiatr.*, 1967, *17*, 751–54.

KEELER, M. H., Marihuana induced hallucinations. *Diseases of the Nervous System*, 1968, *29*, 314–15.

KEITH-SPIEGEL, PATRICIA, and D. E. SPIEGEL, Affective states of patients immediately preceding suicide. *J. Psychiatric Res.*, 1967, *5*, 89–93.

KENNEDY, J. A., and H. BOKST, Emotions and the outcome of cardiac surgery. *Bull. New York Acad. Med.*, 1966, *42*, 811–45.

KENNEDY, W. A., School phobia: rapid treatment of 50 cases. *J. Abnorm. Psychol.*, 1965, *70*, 285–89.

KERRY, R. J., Phobia of outer space. *J. ment. Sci.*, 1960, *106*, 1383–87.

KIGER, R. S., Treating the psychopathic patient in a therapeutic community. *Hospital and Community Psychiatry*, 1967, *15*, 191–96.

KILLAM, R., Psychopharmacological considerations. In *Utopiates*, R. Blum *et al.*, (eds.). New York: Atherton Press, 1964, pp. 118–23.

KINSEY, A. C., W. B. POMEROY, and C. E. MARTIN, *Sexual Behavior in the Human Male*. Philadelphia: W. B. Saunders Co., 1948.

KINSEY, A. C., W. B. POMEROY, and C. E. MARTIN, Concepts of normality and abnormality in sexual behavior. In *Psychosexual Development in Health and Disease*, P. H. Hoch and J. Zubin (eds.). New York: Grune & Stratton, Inc., 1949, pp. 11–32.

KINSEY, A. C., W. B. POMEROY, and C. E. MARTIN, *Sexual Behavior in the Human Female*. Philadelphia: W. B. Saunders Co., 1953.

KISSIN, B., and M. M. GROSS, Drug therapy in alcoholism. *Amer. J. Psychiatr.*, 1968, *125*, 31–41.

KLAW, S., Two weeks in a T-group. *Fortune*, 1961, *64*, 114–17.

KLECHNER, J. H., Personality differences between psychedelic drug users and nonusers. *Psychology*, 1968, *5*, 66–71.

KLERMAN, G., Drugs and Social Values. *Psychiatr. & Soc. Sci. Res.*, 1968, *2*, 2–8.

KNIGHT, J. A., The psychological care of the allergic patient. *Psychosomatics*, 1968, *9*, 160–65.

KOLB, L. C., *Noyes' Modern Clinical Psychiatry* (7th ed.). Philadelphia: W. B. Saunders Co., 1968.

KOPP, S. B., The character structure of sex offenders. *Amer. J. Psychother.*, 1962, *16*, 64–70.

KRASNER, L., The therapist as a social reinforcement machine. In *Research in*

Psychotherapy, H. H. Strupp and L. Luborsky (eds.). Washington: Amer. Psychological Assoc., 1962, pp. 61–94.

KULIK, J. A., K. B. STEIN, and T. R. SARBIN, Dimensions and patterns of adolescent antisocial behavior. *J. consult. & clin. Psychol.*, 1968, *32*, 375–82.

KURILOFF, A. H., and S. ATKINS, T-group for a work team. *J. App. Behavioral Sci.*, 1966, *2*, 63–94.

KURLAND, A. A., S. UNGER, J. W. SHAFFER, and C. SAVAGE, Psychedelic therapy utilizing LSD in the treatment of the alcoholic patient: A preliminary report. *Amer. J. Psychiat.*, 1967, *123*, 1202–9.

LANYON, R. I., Simulation of normal and psychopathic MMPI personality patterns. *J. clin. Psychol.*, 1967, *31*, 94–97.

LARNER, J., and R. TEFFERTELLER, *The Addict in the Street.* New York: Grove Press, Inc., 1964.

LAUGHLIN, H. P., *The Neuroses.* Washington: Butterworths, 1967.

LAZARUS, A. A., The results of behavior therapy in 126 cases of severe neurosis. *Behav. Res. Ther.*, 1963, *1*, 69–79.

LAZARUS, A. A., Learning theory and the treatment of depression. *Behaviour Research and Therapy*, 1968, *6*, 83–89.

LAZARUS, R. S., *Psychological Stress and the Coping Process.* New York: McGraw Hill Book Company, 1966.

LEARY, T., R. METZNER, and R. ALPERT, *The Psychedelic Experience.* New Hyde Park, N. Y.: University Books, 1964.

LERNERT, E. M., The occurrence and sequence of events in the adjustment of families to alcoholism. *Quart. J. Stud. Alcohol*, 1960, *21*, 679–97.

LESTER, D., and L. GREENBERG, Nutrition and the etiology of alcoholism. The effect of sucrose, saccharin and fat on self-selection of ethyl alcohol by rats. *Quart. J. Stud. Alcohol*, 1952, *13*, 553–60.

LEVENTHAL, A. M., Use of a behavioral approach within a traditional psychotherapeutic context: A case study. *J. Abnorm. Psychol.*, 1968, *73*, 178–82.

LEVENTHAL, T., G. WEINBERGER, R. J. STANDLER, and R. P. STEARNS, Therapeutic strategies with school phobics. *Amer. J. Orthopsychiatr.*, 1967, *37*, 64–70.

LEVITT, E. E., *The Psychology of Anxiety.* Indianapolis: The Bobbs-Merrill Co., Inc., 1967.

LEVITT, L., Rehabilitation of narcotics addicts among lower-class teenagers. *Amer. J. Orthopsychiatr.*, 1968, *38*, 56–62.

LEVY, N. J., The use of drugs by teenagers for sanctuary and illusion. *Amer. J. Psychoanal.*, 1968, *28*, 48–58.

LEVY, R. I., The psychodynamic functions of alcohol. *Quart. J. Stud. Alcohol*, 1958, *19*, 649–59.

LIBERMAN, R., Aversive conditioning of drug addicts: A pilot study. *Behaviour Research and Therapy*, 1968, *6*, 229–31.

LIDZ, T., General concepts of psychosomatic medicine. In *American Handbook of Psychiatry*, S. Arieti (ed.). New York: Basic Books, Inc., Publishers, 1959, 647–58.

LIEF, H. I., and D. M. REED, Normal psychosexual functioning. In *Psychiatry*, A. M. Freedman and H. I. Kaplan (eds.). Baltimore, Md.: Williams and Wilkins, 1967, pp. 258–65.

LORAND, S., *Clinical Studies in Psychoanalysis*. New York: International Universities Press, 1950.

LORAND, S., and H. I. SCHNEER, Sexual deviations. III: Fetishism, Transvestitism, Masochism, Sadism, Exhibitionism, Voyeurism, Incest, Pedophilia, and Bestiality. In *Psychiatry*, A. M. Freedman and H. I. Kaplan (eds.). Baltimore: Williams and Wilkins, 1967, pp. 977–88.

LOURIA, D., *Nightmare Drugs*. New York: Pocket Books, 1966.

LOURIA, D. B., Current concepts: Lysergic acid diethylamide. *New England J. of Medicine*, 1968, *278*, 435–38.

LUKIANOWICZ, N., Two cases of transvestism. *Psychiat. Quart.*, 1960, *34*, 517–37.

LYKKEN, D. T., A study of anxiety in sociopathic personality. *J. soc. Psych.*, 1957, *55*, 6–10.

MADDOX, G. L., Drinking among Negroes: Inferences from the drinking patterns of selected Negro male collegians. *J. of Health & Social Behavior*, 1968, *9*, 114–20.

MAHABIR, W., History of the psychedelic drug experience. *Canadian Psychiatric Association Journal*, 1968, *13*, 189–90.

MASSERMAN, J. H., *Dynamic Psychiatry*. Philadelphia: W. B. Saunders Co., 1946.

MARGOLIS, M., The mother-child relationship in bronchial asthma. *J. abnorm. soc. Psychol.*, 1961, *63*, 360–87.

MARKS, I. M., Aversion therapy. *Brit. J. Med. Psychol.*, 1968, *41*, 47–52.

MARTIN, AGNES J., A case of homosexuality and personality disorder in a man of 36 treated by LSD and resolved within two months. *Psychotherapy and Psychosomatics*, 1967, *15*, 44.

MARTIN, J. M., and J. P. FITZPATRICK, *Delinquent Behavior*. New York: Random House, Inc., 1964.

MASTERS, R. E. (ed.), *Sexual Self-Stimulation*. Los Angeles, Calif.: Sherbourne Press, 1967.

MASTERS, R. E. L., and JEAN HOUSTON, *The Varieties of Psychedelic Experience*. New York: Holt, Rinehart, and Winston, Inc., 1966.

MATZA, D., *Delinquency and Drift*. New York: John Wiley & Sons, Inc., 1965.

MAYFIELD, D. G., Psychopharmacology of alcohol: I. Affective change with intoxication, drinking behavior and affective state. *J. nerv. & ment. dis.*, 1968, *146*, 314–21.

MAYFIELD, D. G., Psychopharmacology of alcohol: II. Affective tolerance in alcohol intoxication. *J. nerv. & ment. dis.*, 1968, *146*, 322–27.

MAYFIELD, D., and D. ALLEN, Alcohol and affect: A psychopharmacological study. *Amer. J. Psychiat.*, 1967, *123*, 1346–51.

McCORD, W., and JOAN McCORD, *Psychopathy and Delinquency*. New York: Grune & Stratton, Inc., 1956.

McCORD, W., JOAN McCORD, and J. GUDEMAN, Some current theories of alcoholism. A longitudinal evaluation. *Quart. J. Stud. Alcohol*, 1959, *20*, 727–49.

McGuire, R. J., J. M. Carlisle, and B. G. Young, Sexual deviation as conditioned behaviors: A hypothesis. *Behavior Research and Therapy*, 1965, *2*, 185–90.

McNeil, E. B., Psychology and aggression. *J. Conflict Resolution*, 1959, *3*, 195–293.

McNeil, E. B., *The Quiet Furies*. Englewood Cliffs, N.J.: Prentice-Hall, Inc., 1967.

Meissner, W. W., Family dynamics and psychosomatic processes. *Family Process*, 1966, *5*, 142–61.

Menaker, T., Anxiety about drinking in alcoholics. *J. Abnorm. Psych.*, 1967, *72*, 43–49.

Mendelson, M., Neurotic depressive reaction. In *Psychiatry*, A. M. Freedman and H. I. Kaplan (eds.). Baltimore: Williams and Wilkins, 1967, pp. 928–36.

Mendelson, M., Psychological aspects of obesity. *Int. J. Psychiat.*, 1966, *2*, 599–610.

Menninger, K., *Man Against Himself*. New York: Basic Books, Inc., Publishers, 1938.

Miall, W. E., and P. D. Oldham, The hereditary factor in arterial blood pressure. *Brit. Med. Journal*, 1963, *1*, 75–80.

Michaels, J. J., Character structure and character disorders. In *American Handbook of Psychiatry*, S. Arieti (ed.). New York: Basic Books, Inc., Publishers, 1959, 353–77.

Miller, M. H., Neurosis, psychosis, and the borderline states. In *Psychiatry*, A. M. Freedman and H. I. Kaplan (eds.). Baltimore: Williams and Wilkins, 1967, pp. 589–92.

Miller, P. M., J. B. Bradley, R. S. Gross, and G. Wood, Review of homosexuality research (1960–1966) and some implications for treatment. *Psychotherapy: Theory, Research, and Practice*, 1968, *5*, 3–6.

Mohr, J. W., R. E. Turner, and M. B. Jerry, *Pedophilia and Exhibitionism*. Toronto: Univer. of Toronto Press, 1964.

Montagu, A., Chromosomes and crime. *Psychology Today*, 1968, *2*, 43–49.

Mordhoff, A. M., and O. A. Parsons, The coronary personality: A critique. *Psychosomatic Medicine*, 1967, *29*, 1–12.

Mulder, D. W., and A. J. D. Dale, Brain syndromes associated with infection. In *Psychiatry*, A. M. Freedman and H. I. Kaplan (eds.). Baltimore, Md.: Williams and Wilkins, 1967, pp. 775–86.

Murray, J. B., Drug addiction. *J. general Psychol.*, 1967, *77*, 41–68.

National Training Laboratories, *21st Annual Summer Laboratories*. Washington, D.C., 1967.

Nagler, S. H., The mind-body problem. In *Psychiatry*, A. M. Freedman and H. I. Kaplan (eds.). Baltimore, Md.: Williams and Wilkins Co., 1967, pp. 1037–39.

NEMIAH, J. C., Conversion reaction. In *Psychiatry*, A. M. Freedman and H. I. Kaplan (eds.). Baltimore, Md.: Williams and Wilkins, 1967, pp. 870–85.

NIELSON, J., The XYY syndrome in a mental hospital. *Brit. J. Criminology*, 1968, *8*, 186–203.

NIELSON, J., URSULA FREDERICK, and T. TSUBOI, Chromosome abnormalities and psychotropic drugs. *Nature*, 1968, *218*, 488–89.

NIELSON, P. E., A study in transsexualism. *Psychiat. Quart.*, 1960, *34*, 203–35.

NORTON, W. A., The marihuana habit: Some observations of a small group of users. *Canadian Psychiatric Association Journal*, 1968, *13*, 163–73.

OLIVER, W. A., and D. L. MOSHER, Psychopathology and gilt in heterosexual and subgroups of homosexual reformatory inmates. *J. abnorm. Psychol.*, 1968, *73*, 323–29.

OLSEN, I. A., and H. S. COLEMAN, Treatment of school phobia as a case of separation anxiety. *Psychology in the Schools*, 1967, *4*, 151–54.

O'NEAL, P., L. N. ROBINS, L. KING, and J. SCHAEFER, Parental deviance and the genesis of sociopathic personality. *Amer. J. Psychiat.*, 1962, *118*, 1114–24.

OPLER, M. K., *Culture and Social Psychiatry*. New York: Atherton Press, 1967.

PACHT, A. R., S. L. HALLECK, and J. C. EHRMANN, Diagnosis and treatment of the sex offender: a nine-year study. *Amer. J. Psychiat.*, 1962, *118*, 802–8.

PAINTING, D. H., The performance of psychopathic individuals under conditions of positive and negative partial reinforcement. *J. abnorm. soc. Psychol.*, 1961, *62*, 353–55.

PANTON, J. H., A new MMPI scale for identification of homosexuality. *J. clin. Psych.*, 1960, *16*, 17–20.

PATTISON, E. M., L. A. BISHOP, and A. S. LINSKY, Changes in public attitudes on narcotic addiction. *Amer. J. Psychiatr.*, 1968, *125*, 160–67.

PAUL, G. L., *Insight Versus Desensitization in Psychotherapy: An Experiment in Anxiety Reduction*. Stanford, Calif.: Stanford University Press, 1966.

PEARLMAN, S., Drug use and experience in an urban college population. *Amer. J. Orthopsychiat.*, 1967, *37*, 297–99.

PERVIN, L. A., Some questions concerning illicit use of drugs on the campus. *Amer. J. Orthopsychiatr.*, 1967, *37*, 299.

PESCOR, M. J., A comparative study of male and female drug addicts. *Amer. J. Psychiatry*, 1944, *100*, 771–74.

PICKERING, F., Hyperpiesis: High blood pressure without evident cause— essential hypertension. *Brit. Med. J.*, 1965, *2*, 959–68.

PITTS, F. N., The biochemistry of anxiety. 1969, *220*, 69–75.

POFFENBURGER, R. S., P. A. WOLF, J. NOTKIN, and M. C. THORNE, Chronic disease in former college students. I. Early precursors of fatal coronary disease. *Amer. J. Epidemiology*, 1966, *83*, 314–28.

POKORNY, A. D., Myths about suicide. In *Suicidal Behaviors: Diagnosis and Management*, H. L. P. Resnick (ed.). Boston: Little, Brown, and Company, 1968, pp. 57–72.

POKORNY, A. D., B. A. MILLER, and S. E. CLEVELAND, Response to treatment of alcoholism: a follow-up study. *Quart. J. Stud. in Alcohol*, 1968, *29*, 364–81.

QUINN, J. T., and ROSALIND HENBEST, Partial failure of generalization in alcoholics following aversion therapy. *Quart. J. Stud. Alcohol*, 1967, *28*, 70–75.

RACHMAN, S., Sexual disorders and behavior therapy. *Amer. J. Psychiatr.*, 1961, *118*, 235–40.

RAMSAY, R. W., and V. vanVELZEN, Behaviour therapy for sexual perversions. *Behaviour Research and Therapy*, 1968, *6*, 233.

RAYMOND, M. J., Case of fetishism treated by aversion therapy. *Brit. Med. J.*, 1956, *2*, 854–56.

REES, L., The role of emotional and allergic factors in hay fever. *Psychosomatic Research*, 1959, *3*, 234–41.

REDLICH, F. C., and D. X. FREEDMAN, *The Theory and Practice of Psychiatry*. New York: Basic Books, Inc., Publishers, 1966.

REICH, W., *Character Analysis* (2nd ed.). New York: Orgone Inst. Press, 1945.

REIK, T., *Masochism in Modern Man*. New York: Farrar and Rinehart, 1941.

REINHART, R. F., The flyer who fails: an adult situational reaction. *Amer. J. Psychiatr.*, 1967, *124*, 740–44.

REISER, M. F., Cardiovascular disorders. In *Psychiatry*, A. M. Freedman and H. I. Kaplan (eds.). Baltimore, Md.: Williams and Wilkins, 1967, pp. 1064–67.

REISER, M. F., and H. BOKST, Psychology of cardiovascular disorders. In *American Handbook of Psychiatry*, S. Arieti (ed.). New York: Basic Books, Inc., Publishers, 1959, pp. 659–77.

RESNIK, H. L. P. (ed.), *Suicidial Behaviors: Diagnosis and Management*. Boston: Little, Brown, and Company, 1968.

REVITCH, E., and ROSALEE G. WEISS, The pedophiliac offender. *Dis. nerv. Sys.*, 1962, *23*, 73–78.

RIESMAN, D., with R. DENNY, and N. GLAZER, *The Lonely Crowd*. New Haven: Yale Univer. Press, 1950.

RITCHIE, G. G., The use of hypnosis in a case of exhibitionism. *Psychotherapy: Theory, Research and Practice*, 1968, *5*, 40–43.

ROBINS, E., Antisocial and dysocial personality disorders. In *Psychiatry*, A. M. Freedman and H. I. Kaplan (eds.). Baltimore, Md.: Williams and Wilkins, 1967, pp. 951–58.

ROBINS, L. N., *Deviant Children Grown Up: A Sociological and Psychiatric Study of Sociopathic Personality*. Baltimore, Md.: Williams and Wilkins, 1966.

ROSEN, E., and I. GREGORY, *Abnormal Psychology*. Philadelphia: W. B. Saunders Co., 1965.

ROSEN, H., and J. FRANK, Negroes in psychotherapy. *Amer. J. Psychiatr.*, 1962, *119*, 456–60.

ROSENBERG, C. M., Complications of obsessional neurosis. *Brit. J. Psychiatr.*, 1968, *114*, 477–78.

ROSENKRANTZ, P., SUSAN VOGEL, HELEN BEE, INGE BROVERMAN, and D. M. BROVERMAN, Sex-role stereotypes and self-concepts in college students. *J. consult. & clin. Psychol.*, 1968, *32*, 287–95.

RUBIN, R. D., Treatment of obsessions by conditioned inhibition. *Conditioned Reflex*, 1967, *2*, 167–68.

SANDLER, S. A., Somnambulism in the Armed Forces. *Ment. Hygiene*, 1945, *29*, 236–47.

SANFORD, P., Psychology and the mental health movement. *Amer. Psychol.*, 1958, *13*, 80–85.

SANFORD, N., Personality and patterns of alcohol consumption. *J. consult. & clin. Psychol.*, 1968, *32*, 13–17.

SARGANT, W., and E. SLATER, *An introduction to physical methods of treatment in psychiatry*. Edinburgh: Livingstone, 1954.

SHAPIRO, A. K., A contribution to a history of the placebo effect. *Behav. Sci.*, 1960, *5*, 109–35.

SHAPIRO, D., *Neurotic Styles*. New York: Basic Books, Inc., Publishers, 1965.

SHAROFF, R. L., Sedatives. In *Psychiatry*, A. M. Freedman and H. I. Kaplan (eds.). Baltimore, Md.: Williams and Wilkins, 1967, pp. 1275–77.

SILVERMAN, CHARLOTTE, The epidemiology of depression: A review. *Amer. J. Psychiatr.*, 1968, *124*, 883–91.

SILVERMAN, D., The electroencephalograph and therapy of criminal psychopaths. *J. Crim. Psychopathol.*, 1944, *5*, 439–66.

SIMON, W., and J. H. GAGNON, Femininity in the lesbian community. *Social Problems*, 1967, *15*, 212–21.

SKAKKABAEK, N. E., J. PHILIP, and O. RAFAELSON, LSD in mice: Abnormalities in mitotic chromosomes. *Science*, 1968, *160*, 1246–48.

SOLOMON, D. (ed.), *LSD: The Consciousness-Expanding Drug*. New York: G. P. Putnam's Sons, 1964.

SOLOMON, D. (ed.), *The Marihuana Papers*. Indianapolis: The Bobbs-Merrill Co., Inc., 1966.

SPIELBERGER, C. D., Theory and research on anxiety. In *Anxiety and Behavior*, C. D. Spielberger (ed.). New York: Academic Press, Inc., 1966.

STAFFORD, P. G., and B. H. GOLIGHTLY, *LSD the Problem-Solving Psychedelic*. New York: Award Books, 1967.

STAMPFL, T. G., and D. J. LEVIS, Essentials of implosive therapy: A learning-theory-based psychodynamic behavioral therapy. *J. Abnorm. Psychol.*, 1967, *72*, 496–503.

STERNBACH, A., Object loss and depression. *Arch. Gen. Psychiatr.*, 1965, *12*, 114–51.

STERNBACH, R. A., *Principles of Psychophysiology*. New York: Academic Press, Inc., 1966.

STOLLER, R. J., *Sex and Gender*. New York: Science House, 1968.

STONE, A. A., and H. M. SHEIN, Psychotherapy of the hospitalized suicidal patient. *Amer. J. Psychotherapy*, 1968, *22*, 15–25.

STORM, T., and R. G. SMART, Dissociation: A possible explanation of some features of alcoholism, and implications for its treatment. *Quart. J. Stud. Alcohol.*, 1965, *26*, 111–15.

STOTT, D. H., Evidence for a congenital factor in maladjustment and delinquency. *Amer. J. Psychiat.*, 1962, *118*, 781–84.

STUBBLEFIELD, R. L., Antisocial and dyssocial reactions. In *Psychiatry*, A. M. Freedman and H. I. Kaplan (eds.). Baltimore, Md.: Williams and Wilkins, 1967, pp. 1420–24.

SUCHMAN, E. A., The "hang-loose" ethic and the spirit of drug use. *J. of Health and Social Behavior*, 1968, *9*, 146–55.

SWENSON, W. M., and B. P. GRIMES, Characteristics of sex offenders admitted to a Minnesota state hospital for pre-sentence psychiatric investigation. *Psychiat. Quart. Suppl.*, 1958, *32*, 110–23.

SZASZ, T. S., The myth of mental illness. *Amer. Psychol.*, 1960, *15*, 113–18.

TEICHER, J. D., Patterns and trait disturbances. In *Psychiatry*, A. M. Freedman and H. I. Kaplan (eds.). Baltimore, Md.: Williams and Wilkins, 1967, pp. 1414–20.

TELFER, MARY A., D. BAKER, G. R. CLARK, and C. E. RICHARDSON, Incidence of gross chromosomal errors among tall criminal American males. *Science*, 1968, *159*, 1249–50.

THIGPEN, C. H., and H. M. CLECKLEY, *The Three Faces of Eve*. New York: McGraw-Hill Book Company, 1957.

THORNE, F. C., The etiology of sociopathic reactions. *Amer. J. Psychother.*, 1959, *13*, 319–30.

TOMSOVIC, M., Hospitalized alcoholic patients: I. A two-year study of medical, social, and psychological characteristics. *Hospital and Community Psychiatry*, 1968, *19*, 197–203.

TREISMAN, M., Mind, body, and behavior: Control systems and their disturbances. In *Foundations of Abnormal Psychology*, P. London and D. Rosenhan (eds.). New York: Holt, Rinehart and Winston, Inc., 1968, pp. 460–518.

TURNBULL, J. W., Asthma conceived as a learned response. *J. psychosom. Res.*, 1962, *6*, 59–70.

WAHL, C. W. (ed.), *Sexual Problems: Diagnosis and Treatment in Medical Practice*. New York: Free Press of Glencoe, Inc., 1967.

WAITE, R. R., The Negro patient and clinical theory. *J. consult. and clin. Psychol.*, 1968, *32*, 427–33.

WARDROP, K. R., Delinquent teenage types. *Brit. J. Criminol.*, 1967, *7*, 371–80.

WATKINS, J. G., Psychotherapeutic methods. In *Handbook of Clinical Psychology*, B. B. Wolman (ed.). New York: McGraw-Hill Book Company, 1965, pp. 1143–67.

WEGROCKI, H. J., Validity of the concept of psychopathic personality. *Arch. crim. Psychodyn.*, 1961, *4*, 789–97.

WEINBERG, S. K., *Society and Personality Disorders*. Englewood Cliffs, N.J.: Prentice-Hall, Inc., 1952.

WEISS, E., and O. S. ENGLISH, *Psychosomatic Medicine*. Philadelphia: W. B. Saunders Co., 1957.

WEISS, J. M. A., The suicidal patient. In *American Handbook of Psychiatry*, S. Arieti (ed.). New York: Basic Books, Inc., Publishers, 1966, pp. 115–30.

WEITZENHOFFER, A. M., *Hypnotism: Objective Study in Suggestibility*. New York: John Wiley & Sons, Inc., 1953.

WEST, L. J., Dissociative reaction. In *Psychiatry*, A. M. Freedman and H. I. Kaplan (eds.). Baltimore, Md.: Williams and Wilkins, 1967, pp. 885–99.

WHALEN, THELMA, Wives of alcoholics. Four types observed in family service agency. *Quart. J. Stud. Alcohol*, 1953, *14*, 632–41.

WHITE, R. W., *The Abnormal Personality*. New York: The Ronald Press Company, 1964.

WHITEHOUSE, F. A., "Cardiacs" without heart disease. *J. Rehabilitation*, 1967, *33*, 14–15.

WICKRAMASEKERA, I., The application of learning theory to the treatment of a case of sexual exhibitionism. *Psychotherapy: Theory, Research, and Practice*, 1968, 5, 108–12.

WIKLER, A., Addictions. I: Opioid addiction. In *Psychiatry*, A. M. Freedman and H. I. Kaplan (eds.). Baltimore, Md.: Williams and Wilkins, 1967, pp. 989–1001.

WILLIAMS, R. J., The etiology of alcoholism: a working hypothesis involving the interplay of hereditary and environmental factors. *Quart. J. Stud. Alcohol*, 1947, 7, 567–87.

WILLIAMS, R. J., *Alcoholism: the nutritional approach*. Austin: Univer. of Texas Press, 1959.

WILSON, A., and F. J. SMITH, Counterconditioning therapy using free association: a pilot study. *J. Abnorm. Psychol.*, 1968, 73, 474–78.

WIRT, R. D., P. F. BRIGGS, and J. GOLDEN, Delinquency prone personalities. III: The sociopathic personality: treatment. *Minnesota Med.*, 1962, 45, 289–95.

WITTHOWER, E. D., and K. L. WHITE, Psychophysiologic aspects of respiratory disorders. In *American Handbook of Psychiatry*, S. Arieti (ed.). New York: Basic Books, Inc., Publishers, 1959, pp. 690–707.

WITZIG, J. S., The group treatment of male exhibitionists. *Amer. J. Psychiatry*, 1968, *125*, 179–85.

WOLF, S., and H. G. WOLFF, *Headaches: their nature and treatment*. Boston: Little, Brown, and Company, 1953.

The Wolfenden Report: Report of the Committee on Homosexual Offenses and Prostitution. New York: Stein and Day, 1963.

WOLMAN, B. B., Clinical psychology and the philosophy of Science. In *Handbook of Clinical Psychology*, B. B. Wolman (ed.). New York: McGraw-Hill Book Company, 1965.

WOLPE, J., *Psychotherapy by reciprocal inhibition*. Stanford: Stanford Univer. Press, 1958.

WOLPE, J., Phobic reactions and behavior therapy. *Conditional Reflex*, 1967, 2, 162.

YABLONSKY, L., Where is science taking us? *Saturday Rev.*, 1963, *46*, 54–56.

YABLONSKY, L., *Synanon: The Tunnel Back*. Baltimore, Md.: Penguin Books, Inc., 1967.

ZWERDLING, I., and M. ROSENBAUM, Alcoholic addiction and personality (nonpsychotic conditions). In *American Handbook of Psychiatry*, S. Arieti (ed.). New York: Basic Books, Inc., Publishers, 1959, pp. 623–44.

Index